Kimitaka Kaga · Arnold Starr (Eds.)

Neuropathies of the Auditory and Vestibular Eighth Cranial Nerves

Kimitaka Kaga · Arnold Starr
Editors

Neuropathies of the Auditory and Vestibular Eighth Cranial Nerves

Springer

Kimitaka Kaga, M.D., Ph.D.
Emeritus Professor, The University of Tokyo
Director, National Institute of Sensory Organs
National Tokyo Medical Center
2-5-1 Higashigaoka, Meguro-ku, Tokyo 152-8902, Japan

Arnold Starr, M.D.
Professor
Department of Neurology and Neurobiology
University of California Irvine
Irvine, CA 92717, USA

ISBN 978-4-431-99804-4
e-ISBN 978-4-431-09433-3

Springer is a part of Springer Science+Business Media
springer.com

Printed in Japan

Printed on acid-free paper

Preface

The International Mini-Symposium on Auditory and Vestibular Neuropathy (Auditory Nerve Disease) was held on March 3, 2007, at the University of Tokyo, Japan. The symposium was planned to commemorate my new departure from the University of Tokyo to the National Institute of Sensory Organs. Guest speakers from the United States, Australia, Korea, and Japan presented papers that focused on history, gene, pathophysiology, analysis, perception, sound localization, cochlear implants, and balance for auditory and vestibular neuropathy, with up-to-date information and knowledge. Altogether, there were many important presentations about this new disease, which was first reported by Kaga K et al and Starr A et al in 1996. There are many unsolved issues such as gene location, site of pathology, and the effect of cochlear implants. In the last 10 years, hearing screening of newborns has been introduced in many countries, and auditory neuropathy is paid much more attention because of the increase in new findings. In this international mini-symposium, in addition to auditory neuropathy, vestibular neuropathy in particular was discussed because of the simultaneous existence of both auditory and vestibular issues.

This book provides up-to-date information and knowledge on the neuropathy of auditory and vestibular eighth nerves VIII. The title for the book was suggested by Prof. Arnold Starr as one that would cover the entire range of topics. I am hopeful that, with this book, readers can gain insight into the new disease entity, auditory and vestibular neuropathy.

I would like to acknowledge, with gratitude, that this publication was financially supported in part by the alumni association of the Department of Otolaryngology, Faculty of Medicine, University of Tokyo, and by the Society for the Promotion of Oto-Rhino-Laryngology.

Kimitaka Kaga, M.D., Ph.D.
Director, National Institute of Sensory Organs
Tokyo Medical Center
Emeritus Professor, The University of Tokyo

Contents

Contributors

Yusuke Akamatsu
Department of Otolaryngology, and Head and Neck Surgery, The University of Tokyo, Tokyo, Japan

Swee T. Aw
Neurology Department, Royal Prince Alfred Hospital, Sydney, NSW, Australia

Ian S. Curthoys
Neurology Department, Royal Prince Alfred Hospital, Sydney, NSW, Australia

Shouichiro Fukuda
Okayama Kanaria Gakuen, Okayama, Japan

Kunihiro Fukushima
Department of Otolaryngology Head and Neck Surgery, Okayama University Postgraduate School of Medicine, Dentistry and Pharmaceutical Science, Okayama, Japan

William P.R. Gibson
Department of Surgery, University of Sydney, Sydney, NSW, Australia

G. Michael Halmagyi
Neurology Department, Royal Prince Alfred Hospital, Sydney, NSW, Australia

Masumi Inagaki
Department of Developmental Disorders, National Institute of Mental Health, National Center of Neurology and Psychiatry (NCNP), Tokyo, Japan

Kenji Itoh
Department of Sensory and Motor Neuroscience, The University of Tokyo School of Medicine, Tokyo, Japan

Sung-Wook Jeong
Department of Otolaryngology—Head and Neck Surgery, College of Medicine, Dong-A University, Busan, Korea

Yulian Jin
National Institute of Sensory Organs, National Tokyo Medical Center, Tokyo, Japan

Kimitaka Kaga
National Institute of Sensory Organs, National Tokyo Medical Center, Tokyo, Japan

Makiko Kaga
Department of Developmental Disorders, National Institute of Mental Health, National Center of Neurology and Psychiatry (NCNP), Tokyo, Japan

Shin Kariya
Department of Otolaryngology Head and Neck Surgery, Okayama University Postgraduate School of Medicine, Dentistry and Pharmaceutical Science, Okayama, Japan

Yuko Kataoka
Department of Otolaryngology Head and Neck Surgery, Okayama University Postgraduate School of Medicine, Dentistry and Pharmaceutical Science, Okayama, Japan

Akihiro Kawasaki
Department of Otolaryngology Head and Neck Surgery, Okayama University Postgraduate School of Medicine, Dentistry and Pharmaceutical Science, Okayama, Japan

Ken Kazahaya
Division of Pediatric Otolaryngology, The Children's Hospital of Philadelphia, Philadelphia, PA, USA
Department of Otolaryngology: Head and Neck Surgery, University of Pennsylvania School of Medicine, Philadelphia, PA, USA

Lee-Suk Kim
Department of Otolaryngology—Head and Neck Surgery, College of Medicine, Dong-A University, Busan, Korea

Kaori Kon
Department of Developmental Disorders, National Institute of Mental Health, National Center of Neurology and Psychiatry (NCNP), Tokyo, Japan

Shozo Kuroki
Department of Sensory and Motor Neuroscience, The University of Tokyo School of Medicine, Tokyo, Japan

Yukihide Maeda
Department of Otolaryngology Head and Neck Surgery, Okayama University Postgraduate School of Medicine, Dentistry and Pharmaceutical Science, Okayama, Japan

Roger R. Marsh
Center for Childhood Communication, and Division of Pediatric Otolaryngology, The Children's Hospital of Philadelphia, Philadelphia, PA, USA

Tatsuo Matsunaga
Laboratory of Auditory Disorders, National Institute of Sensory Organs, National Tokyo Medical Center, Tokyo, Japan

Catherine M. McMahon
Center for Language Sciences, Macquarie University, Sydney, NSW, Australia

Toshihisa Murofushi
Department of Otolaryngology, Teikyo University School of Medicine Mizonokuchi Hospital, Kawasaki, Japan

Rie Nagayasu
Department of Otolaryngology Head and Neck Surgery, Okayama University Postgraduate School of Medicine, Dentistry and Pharmaceutical Science, Okayama, Japan

Kazunori Nishizaki
Department of Otolaryngology Head and Neck Surgery, Okayama University Postgraduate School of Medicine, Dentistry and Pharmaceutical Science, Okayama, Japan

Tatsuro Nobutoki
Division of Child Neurology, National Center Hospital, National Center of Neurology and Psychiatry (NCNP), Tokyo, Japan

Robert B. Patuzzi
Department of Physiology, School of Biomedical and Chemical Sciences, University of Western Australia, Perth, WA, Australia

Yuki Saito
Department of Otolaryngology, Tokyo Metropolitan Police Hospital, Tokyo, Japan

Halit Sanli
Sydney Cochlear Implant Centre, Sydney, NSW, Australia

Tunemasa Sato
Department of Otolaryngology, Tokyo Metropolitan Police Hospital, Tokyo, Japan

Sotaro Sekimoto
Department of Sensory and Motor Neuroscience, The University of Tokyo School of Medicine, Tokyo, Japan

Yukiko Shinjo
National Institute of Sensory Organs, National Tokyo Medical Center, Tokyo, Japan

Arnold Starr
Department of Neurology, University of California Irvine, Irvine, CA, USA

Mitsuya Suzuki
Department of Otolaryngology, and Head and Neck Surgery, The University of Tokyo, Tokyo, Japan

Michael J. Todd
Neurology Department, Royal Prince Alfred Hospital, Sydney, NSW, Australia

Naomi Toida
Okayama Kanaria Gakuen, Okayama, Japan

Susumu Tominaga
Department of Otolaryngology Head and Neck Surgery, Okayama University Postgraduate School of Medicine, Dentistry and Pharmaceutical Science, Okayama, Japan

Toshihiro Tsuzuku
Department of Otolaryngology, Teikyo University School of Medicine, Tokyo, Japan

Akira Uno
Department of Developmental Disorders, National Institute of Mental Health, National Center of Neurology and Psychiatry (NCNP), Tokyo, Japan

Konrad P. Weber
Neurology Department, Royal Prince Alfred Hospital, Sydney, NSW, Australia

Tatsuya Yamasoba
Department of Otolaryngology, and Head and Neck Surgery, The University of Tokyo, Tokyo, Japan

Part I
Overview

"Hearing" and Auditory Neuropathy: Lessons from Patients, Physiology, and Genetics

To honor Kimitaka Kaga, scientist-clinician

Arnold Starr

Summary

I review auditory neuropathy (AN), an auditory temporal processing disorder, drawing upon lessons from patients, from temporal bones and peripheral nerves, and from the genetics of the disorder. The auditory temporal processing disorder affects speech comprehension and localization of sounds that can be disabling. Audibility is typically not the majoy problem. The criteria for diagnosis are physiological and include (1) abnormal auditory nerve function reflected by absent or abnormal auditory brainstem responses (ABRs) and (2) normal cochlear outer hair cell functions reflected by cochlear microphonics (CMs) and/or otoacoustic emissions (OAEs). The tests are relatively simple, and the results are typically unambiguous, encouraging the recognition of AN from diverse etiologies. The cochlear sites that are affected include auditory nerve, inner hair cells, or their synapses. Type I AN is a postsynaptic disorder involving both the number and functions of auditory nerves; Type II AN is a presynaptic disorder affecting inner hair cells' ability to form and/or release neurotransmitters. Inherited forms of AN are diverse. Temporal bone studies of postsynaptic forms of AN show a marked loss of auditory nerve fibers with accompanying demyelination whereas both the number and morphology of inner and outer hair cells are preserved. There are as yet no temporal bone studies of presynaptic forms of AN.

Key words Deafferentation, Neural timing, Genetics, Auditory neuropathy

Introduction

A young, 8-year-old girl with a puzzling hearing disorder was referred to me in 1988 by Manny Don and Yvonne Sininger from the House Ear Research Center. She had normal audiometric pure tone thresholds but impaired speech perception.

Department of Neurology, University of California Irvine, Irvine, CA 92697, USA

doi: 10.1007/978-4-431-09433-3_1,

She was identified as having hearing problems by her teacher when her performance in class declined. She is named, metaphorically, "Eve," as our first patient with "auditory neuropathy." She described her problem as "I can hear but not understand." We studied her in detail for the next 2 years and identified that she had an auditory temporal processing disorder, absent auditory brainstem potentials, and preserved cochlear microphonics, consistent with auditory nerve dysfunction in the presence of normal cochlear receptor hair cells. The article about "Eve" was published in 1991 and needed nine authors to define the condition [1]. Dr. Berlin from the Kresge Hearing Center in New Orleans published a report in 1993 on this same type of hearing disorder and localized the problem to the type I afferent auditory nerve fibers [2]. He organized combining of our efforts and invited our group to come to New Orleans and see some of their patients together. Most of the patients had accompanying neurological disorders that affected their peripheral nerves, and we presumed their auditory nerve was also affected. The exceptions were patients with normal peripheral nerve function, indicating that the dysfunction of the auditory nerve could also reflect a consequence of disorders of inner hair cells and their synapses with auditory nerve. We wrote an article describing their common features succinctly entitled "Auditory Neuropathy" [3].

The unexpected combination of absent or abnormal auditory brainstem responses (ABRs) and normal pure tone audiograms had been noted previously, beginning with Hallowell Davis and S.K. Hirsch, who estimated its incidence was 0.5% in hearing-impaired subjects [4]. Kamitaka Kaga, who is feted in this volume, correctly localized the disorder to the auditory nerve in two elderly patients in 1996 who also had involvement of the vestibular nerves [5].

Auditory neuropathy patients have a wide variety of pure tone hearing loss and in many, speech is impaired out of proportion to the audiometric loss. The finding of absent ABRs when thresholds were elevated to a mild or moderate degree was a paradox because ABRs were being used then, and are still today, as an objective screening test for "hearing." The ABR is more precisely an objective measure of the integrity of function of the auditory nerve and brainstem auditory pathway structures [6]. The information derived from the ABR can provide insights into underlying mechanisms of hearing and its disorders.

The First Lesson: "Time is of the Essence"

The ABR is a measure of brainstem and auditory nerve functions that depends on precise neural encoding of auditory temporal cues. Neurophysiological studies have shown that the neurons in auditory nerve and auditory brainstem structures such as the cochlear nucleus and superior olive are sensitive to microsecond changes of the acoustic signal. The neural code for such temporal events provide signals for such daily processes as speech comprehension and localizing sound sources. The failure to define an ABR in auditory neuropathy (AN) subjects who can hear the clicks may be related to the failure of the auditory nerve to discharge at the same latency to each stimulus so that the averaged neural response cannot be distinguished from the background potentials, known as dys-synchrony We have modeled the effects of such temporal jitter of nerve discharges on the ABRs in the 1991 report describing Eve [1].

We learned what effects impaired auditory neural temporal processing had by examining what these patients could hear and what they could not hear. Eve taught us that rapid time sequences could not be processed: she was impaired on detecting two stimuli presented in rapid sequence. She could not integrate temporal cues presented to each ear, so that localizing signal sources in the environment was deficient. In contrast, intensity discrimination was preserved [1]. My colleague at Irvine, Fan Gang Zeng, made detailed psychoacoustic measures in a number of other AN subjects showing that the common denominator underlying their auditory perceptual deficits is impaired auditory temporal processing [7].

The Second Lesson: "Diagnosis Is Only a Beginning"

The physiological criteria for defining abnormal auditory nerve functions in the presence of preserved receptor activities are a short list [3].

1. Absence or marked abnormality of the ABR, beyond what would be expected for the audiometric threshold elevations.
2. Preserved cochlear receptor functions evidenced by presence of otoacoustic emissions (OAEs) and/or cochlear microphonics (CMs), both generated by outer hair cells. The summating potential (SP), generated primarily by inner hair cells, is of relatively small amplitude and difficult to resolve in the ABR [8].

We also noted that acoustic middle ear muscle reflexes were absent or markedly elevated, and this measure can serve as an adjunct for diagnosing AN [3]. We did not include perceptual measures of temporal processes for diagnosis because cooperation by the subject is required and so many of the patients with AN are infants and children. The identification of these youngsters reflected the widespread use of ABRs and OAEs as objective screening measures of auditory function in the newborn nursery.

AN and its physiological measures can change over time. In approximately one-third of the patients, the disorder progresses to also involve the mechanical properties of cochlear outer hair cells, reflected by the loss of otoacoustic emissions, whereas cochlear microphonics typically persist [9]. Neonates with hypoxia or bilirubinemia can show improvement over time of both ABRs and behavioral measures of hearing. Adults with Guillain–Barré syndrome, an acute immunological disorder, can temporarily lose their hearing as a result of acute demyelination of the auditory nerve [10]. Later in this chapter I discuss adults who are encountered with criteria for AN (absent ABRs and normal otoacoustic emissions) but who are asymptomatic. AN is clearly diverse in both etiology and time-course, and relationship to perceptual disorders requires vigilance to appreciate its dynamic features.

Our appreciation of underlying mechanisms of AN has utilized studies of temporal bones from AN patients after death. At least five temporal bones are examined [11–15]. Three of the earliest temporal bones, studied by Hallpike and Spoendlin, preceded the recognition of AN, but their descriptions of the hearing disorder are compatible with AN. All the patients to date had hereditary neurological disorders affecting peripheral and cranial nerves. Their temporal bones showed marked loss of auditory neural ganglion cells, axons, and dendrites. The inner and outer hair cells were normal in appearance. Some of the remaining auditory nerve fibers show varying degrees of demyelination. Similar changes were found in both affected peripheral and vestibular nerves [13,16], even though there were no clinical symptoms of vestibular nerve involvement [16]. The vestibular neuropathy is "asymptomatic," an alert that auditory neuropathy also can be "asymptomatic". There is a temporal bone study in premature infants with absent ABRs (unfortunately OAEs or CMs were not examined) showing in some a selective loss of inner hair cells without loss of auditory nerves. The incidence of this finding in the 12 temporal bones examined was 25%. As far as I am aware, an isolated loss of inner hair cells is not described in adult temporal bones. The difference between neonates and adults may reflect a particular sensitivity of inner hair cells to anoxia in the developing cochlea [17].

The Third Lesson Is from Genetics: "AN is a Many-Splendored Thing"

AN is similar to other medical conditions by involving multiple etiologies and multiple mechanisms. Genetics provide clear examples of this diversity. I have reviewed the literature (see Table 1) and our own experiences here at Irvine and classified AN. The classification is organized around the synapse that links inner hair cells (presynaptic site) with the auditory nerve (postsynaptic site). Such a model has been successful in defining disorders of neuromuscular function. The classification includes (1) anatomical sites affected (inner hair cell, auditory nerve, their synapse); (2) whether peripheral or optic nerves are involved; (3) type of functions affected (nerve activity, transmitter formation, release, and reuptake, receptor actions); and (4) site of action of the affected gene action (mitochondrial or not). The latter distinction appears to have particular phenotypes involving both optic and auditory nerves accompanying mitochondrial dysfunctions.

The following groupings of AN are proposed:

a. Type I postsynaptic AN: plus vestibular and peripheral neuropathies
b. Type I postsynaptic AN: plus optic nerve disorders accompanying nuclear and mitochondrial mutations affecting mitochondria
c. Type II presynaptic AN: inner hair cell and transmitter disorders
d. AN unspecified: affected sites unknown

Table 1. Genetic varieties of auditory neuropathy (AN)

Groupings	Gene	Inheritance	Sites affected	Other features
Type I: AN postsynaptic: ganglion cells, axons, dendrites:				
With sensory/motor neuropathy (Charcot–Marie–Tooth, CMT)	Nuclear		Neurons Nerves	
i. HSMN-Lom	NDRG1	R	Schwann	Roma
ii. HSMN-myelin protein zero	*MPZ*	D	Axon	
Pathology: Loss of ganglion cells and VIII nerve; hair cells normal				
iii. HSMN-peripheral myelin protein	*PMP22*	R	Schwann	
iv. HSMN-neurofilament light	*NF-L*	D	Axon	Asymptomatic
v. Gap junction protein	*GJB1, 2,*	R	Axon	Connexin
vi. AUNX1	q23-q27.3	X-linked	?	
With optic neuropathy	Nuclear and mitochondrial			Mitochondrial functions
i Optic atrophy 1	*OPA1*	D	Terminals	Nuclear
ii. Leber's optic atrophy	Various			Mitochondria
iii. Friedreich's ataxia	FXN	R	Axons	Variable phenotype
Pathology: Loss of ganglion cells and VIII nerve; hair cells normal				
iv. Multiple systems atrophy	?	R	?	
v. Wolfram 1	WFS1	R	Axons	Variable phenotype
vi. Mohr-Tranebjaerg	*(DDP/TIMM8A*	R	Axons	Variable phenotype
Pathology: Loss of ganglion cells and VIII nerve; hair cells normal				
Auditory neuropathy alone				
i. Perjvakin	DFNB59	R	?	OHC?
ii. AUNA1	13q14–21	D	?	AN young OHC old
Type II AN: presynaptic:				
1. Inner hair cell				
i. Otoferlin	*OTOF*	R	IHC	Temperature sensitive
ii. Gap junction proteins	*GBJ6*	R	IHC	Connexin

OHC, outer hair cells

The Fourth Lesson: "Be Hopeful for AN"

Cochlear implants (CI) work in AN to improve speech perception and psychoacoustic measures of temporal processes [18,19]. Eve has a CI and depends on it to assist lip reading, which has been the major adaptation to her limitations. Eve is a good lip reader and becomes even better when using the implant.

I am of the opinion that learning to hear is lifelong and not restricted to "critical periods." The current trend to implant children with AN during the first year of life so as to be within one of the "critical periods" may not be without flaws. We know that the tests used to diagnose AN can improve in some children [20]. Moreover, adults fulfilling the criteria for AN can be asymptomatic [21] or only symptomatic under certain conditions [22,23]. Such exceptions test the rule that implants should be used in AN without behavioral evidence of impaired auditory temporal processing. The ABR is a brainstem measure and will not reflect brain processes that can adapt to the temporal processing disorder. There are new cortical potential methods of auditory temporal processing that can be used to examine infants as objective measure of cortical processes related to behavioral measures. I suggest that to wait for this evidence is in the best interest of the patient. Observation and new data will help to resolve the issues. As we begin to define the variety of mechanisms of AN, we will have the opportunity to develop appropriate therapies that will be focused and specific for different types of AN.

AN has taught me to listen to my patients. Each one provides unique insights. It is also necessary to make sense of their diversity, to find their common features. Sometimes we do have success, but the real joy is in the process of trying to understand.

This study was supported by Grant #DC 02618 from the National Iustitute on Deafness and Other Communicative Disorders.

References

1. Starr A, McPherson D, Patterson J, et al (1991) Absence of both auditory evoked potentials and auditory percepts dependent on timing cues. Brain 114:1157–1180
2. Berlin CI, Hood LJ, Cecola RP, et al (1993) Does type I afferent neuron dysfunction reveal itself through lack of efferent suppression? Hear Res 65:40–50
3. Starr A, Picton TW, Sininger Y, et al (1996) Auditory neuropathy. Brain 119:741–753
4. Davis H, Hirsh SK (1979) A slow brain stem response for low-frequency audiometry. Audiology 18:445–461
5. Kaga K, Nakamura M, Shinogami M, et al (1996) Auditory nerve disease of both ears revealed by auditory brainstem responses, electrocochleography and otoacoustic emissions. Scand Audiol 25:233–238
6. Starr A (1978) Sensory evoked potentials in clinical disorders of the nervous system. Annu Rev Neurosci 1:103–127
7. Zeng FG, Kong YY, Michalewski HJ, et al (2005) Perceptual consequences of disrupted auditory nerve activity. J Neurophysiol 93:3050–3063

8. Starr A, Sininger Y, Nguyen T, et al (2001) Cochlear receptor (microphonic and summating potentials, otoacoustic emissions) and auditory pathway (auditory brain stem potentials) activity in auditory neuropathy. Ear Hear 22:91–99
9. Sininger Y, Starr A (eds) (2001) Auditory neuropathy. Singular, San Diego
10. Nelson KR, Gilmore RL, Massey A (1988) Acoustic nerve-conduction abnormalities in Guillain-Barre syndrome. Neurology 38:1263–1266
11. Hallpike CS, Harriman DG, Wells CE (1980) A case of afferent neuropathy and deafness. J Laryngol Otol 94:945–964
12. Spoendlin H (1974) Optic cochleovestibular degenerations in hereditary ataxias. II. Temporal bone pathology in two cases of Friedreich's ataxia with vestibulo-cochlear disorders. Brain 97:41–48
13. Starr A, Michalewski HJ, Zeng FG, et al (2003) Pathology and physiology of auditory neuropathy with a novel mutation in the MPZ gene (Tyr145->Ser). Brain 126:1604–1619
14. Starr A (2003) Subspecialization in orthopaedics: is there really too much? J Bone Joint Surg Am 85:1849–1850
15. Bahmad F Jr, Merchant SN, Nadol JB Jr (2007) Otopathology in Mohr-Tranebjaerg syndrome. Laryngoscope 117:1202–1208
16. Fujikawa S, Starr A (2000) Vestibular neuropathy accompanying auditory and peripheral neuropathies. Arch Otolaryngol Head Neck Surg 126:1453–1456
17. Amatuzzi MG, Northrop C, Liberman MC, et al (2001) Selective inner hair cell loss in premature infants and cochlea pathological patterns from neonatal intensive care unit autopsies. Arch Otolaryngol Head Neck Surg 127:629–636
18. Starr A, Isaacson B, Michalewski HJ, et al (2004) A dominantly inherited progressive deafness affecting distal auditory nerve and hair cells. J Assoc Res Otolaryngol 5:411–426
19. Peterson A, Shallop J, Driscoll C, et al (2003) Outcomes of cochlear implantation in children with auditory neuropathy. J Am Acad Audiol 14:188–201
20. Attias J, Raveh E (2007) Transient deafness in young candidates for cochlear implants. Audiol Neurootol 12:325–333
21. Butinar D, Starr A, Zidar J, et al (2008) Auditory nerve is affected in one of two different point mutations of the neurofilament light gene. Clin Neurophysiol 119:367–375
22. Starr A, Sininger Y, Winter M, et al (1998) Transient deafness due to temperature-sensitive auditory neuropathy. Ear Hear 19:169–179
23. Varga R, Avenarius MR, Kelley PM, et al (2006) OTOF mutations revealed by genetic analysis of hearing loss families including a potential temperature sensitive auditory neuropathy allele. J Med Genet 43:576–581

Part II
Pathophysiology and Genetics

Auditory Nerve Disease, New Classification: Auditory and Vestibular Neuropathy

Kimitaka Kaga

Summary

Five of eight patients who were evaluated had auditory nerve disease (AN), with simultaneous hearing and balance problems, and their complaints had not changed over the past few years. Clinical tests of the balance system in these five patients indicated abnormality on the Mann test with eyes closed. Ice water caloric stimulation failed to elicit nystagmus in these patients. Strong rotational testing yielded results consistent with bilaterally impaired function of the horizontal semicircular canals and/or vestibular nerves. In the same five patients, the vestibular-evoked myogenic potential (VEMP) was abolished. It is suggested that the terms "auditory neuropathy only," "auditory-vestibular neuropathy," and "vestibular neuropathy only" in AN could be used to characterize these patients with involvement of only the auditory branch of the VIII cranial nerve in both the auditory and vestibular branches. This usage may help to categorize this disorder more pathophysiologically.

Key words Auditory neuropathy, Vestibular neuropathy, VIII cranial nerve

Introduction

In 1966, Kaga et al. reported a new entity of hearing disorder as "Auditory Nerve Disease" in *Scandinavian Audiology* [1], and Starr et al. reported "Auditory Neuropathy" in *Brain* [2] (Fig. 1). These two different names are considered to refer to the same disease. Their common auditory findings are (1) mild threshold elevation by pure tone audiometry, (2) poor maximum speech discrimination, (3) normal otoacoustic emissions, and (4) absent auditory brainstem response (ABR). Moreover, we found the presence of summating potentials but no compound action potentials in electrocochleography. However, the presence or absence of vestibular problems in these diseases has been controversial.

There is very little information in the literature regarding the involvement, if any, of the vestibular system in auditory nerve disease or auditory neuropathy (AN).

National Institute of Sensory Organs, National Tokyo Medical Center, 2-5-1 Higashigaoka, Meguro-ku, Tokyo 152-8902, Japan

doi: 10.1007/978-4-431-09433-3_2, © Springer 2009

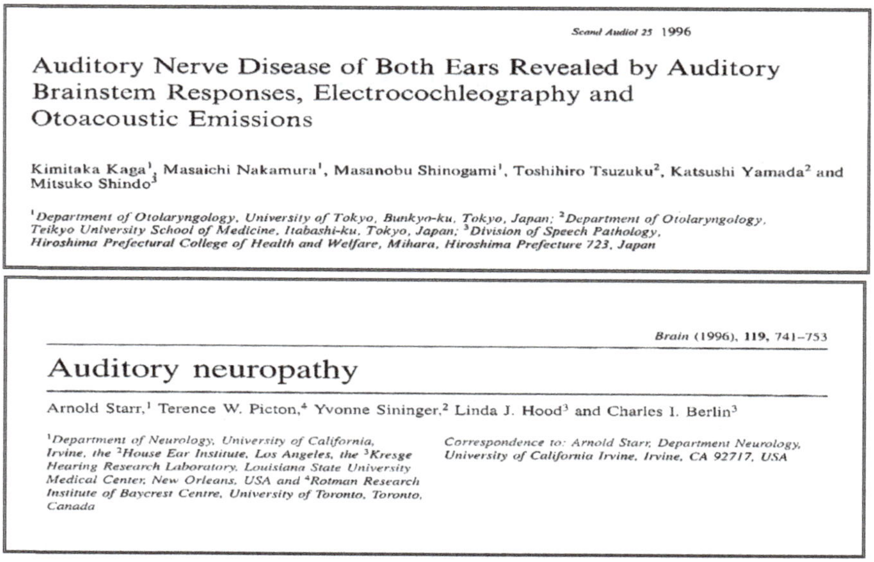
Scand Audiol 25 1996

Auditory Nerve Disease of Both Ears Revealed by Auditory Brainstem Responses, Electrocochleography and Otoacoustic Emissions

Kimitaka Kaga[1], Masaichi Nakamura[1], Masanobu Shinogami[1], Toshihiro Tsuzuku[2], Katsushi Yamada[2] and Mitsuko Shindo[3]

[1]Department of Otolaryngology, University of Tokyo, Bunkyo-ku, Tokyo, Japan; [2]Department of Otolaryngology, Teikyo University School of Medicine, Itabashi-ku, Tokyo, Japan; [3]Division of Speech Pathology, Hiroshima Prefectural College of Health and Welfare, Mihara, Hiroshima Prefecture 723, Japan

Brain (1996), 119, 741–753

Auditory neuropathy

Arnold Starr,[1] Terence W. Picton,[4] Yvonne Sininger,[2] Linda J. Hood[3] and Charles I. Berlin[3]

[1]Department of Neurology, University of California, Irvine, the [2]House Ear Institute, Los Angeles, the [3]Kresge Hearing Research Laboratory, Louisiana State University Medical Center, New Orleans, USA and [4]Rotman Research Institute of Baycrest Centre, University of Toronto, Toronto, Canada

Correspondence to: Arnold Starr, Department Neurology, University of California Irvine, Irvine, CA 92717, USA

Fig. 1. The first two reports in 1996

Table 1. Profile of patients

Case No.	Age (yrs.)	Onset (yrs.)	Remark
1	16	6	Cerebral infarction
2	22	11	Blindness
3	22	15	Spinocerebellar ataxia
4	27	11	
5	31	6	Viral cerebellitis
6	57	15	
7	60	35	
8	72	Teenager	

To contribute to the physiological and psychophysical knowledge of AN, we report here our auditory and vestibular system assessment of our patients diagnosed with this disorder.

Patients

Eight patients were evaluated in this study (16M, 22M, 28F, 30F, 31M, 57F, 61F, 72F; the number is years of age, and M and F mean male or female, respectively; Table 1). All patients complained of a hearing problem and poor discrimination of speech on the telephone and all were subsequently found to have preserved oto-acoustic emissions (OAEs), preserved electrocochleograms (ECochGs), and absent or severely distorted ABRs. In addition, most patients complained of equilibrium problems. There were no consistent findings in their past medical histories or familial hearing disorders or consanguineous marriage in the pedigree.

Methods

Auditory Function Tests

All patients underwent standard pure tone audiometry, speech discrimination test, and the token test.

Auditory physiological tests: distortion product otoacoustic emissions (DPOAE) were recorded and analyzed. ABRs to click stimuli were recorded. ECochGs to click stimuli were recorded by extratympanic electrodes placed on the eardrum.

Vestibular Function Tests

The Romberg and Mann tests with eyes open and closed were scored for each patient.

All patients underwent an electronystagmography (ENG) test battery.

Ice water (2 cm^3) caloric testing was performed to irrigate the external auditory meatus to induce a thermal gradient across the lateral semicircular canal. The damped-rotation test was added for patients in cases of loss of caloric nystagmus (EVAR). Vestibular-evoked myogenic potentials (VEMP) were recorded. The ear was stimulated with the sternocleidomastoid muscle to click (SCM). Responses to 200 clicks at an intensity of 95 dB nHL, presented at 5 Hz, were recorded in 100-ms intervals over a bandpass of 20–2000 Hz.

Results

Auditory Assessment Results

All patients had a low-frequency loss with a rising slope pattern, the severity of which ranged from mild to moderate (Fig. 2). Speech discrimination scores were markedly abnormal in all patients despite the mild-to-moderate elevation of the pure tone audiograms, suggesting retrocochlear pathology (Fig. 3).

All eight patients had demonstrated normal DPOAEs in both ears, but their ABRs were essentially abolished, and ECochGs were also abolished but summating potentials were preserved (Fig. 4). In Fig. 5, five auditory tests of case 1 are shown.

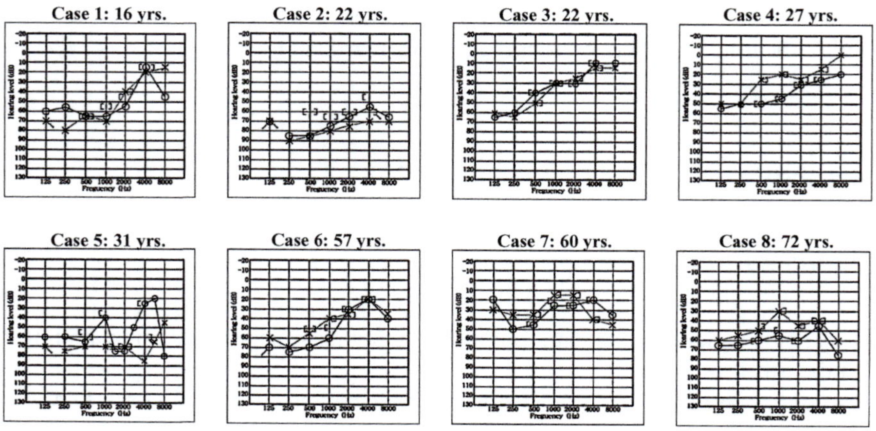

Fig. 2. Pure tone audiograms. All audiograms show a low-frequency loss with a rising slopes pattern, the severity of which ranged from mild to moderate

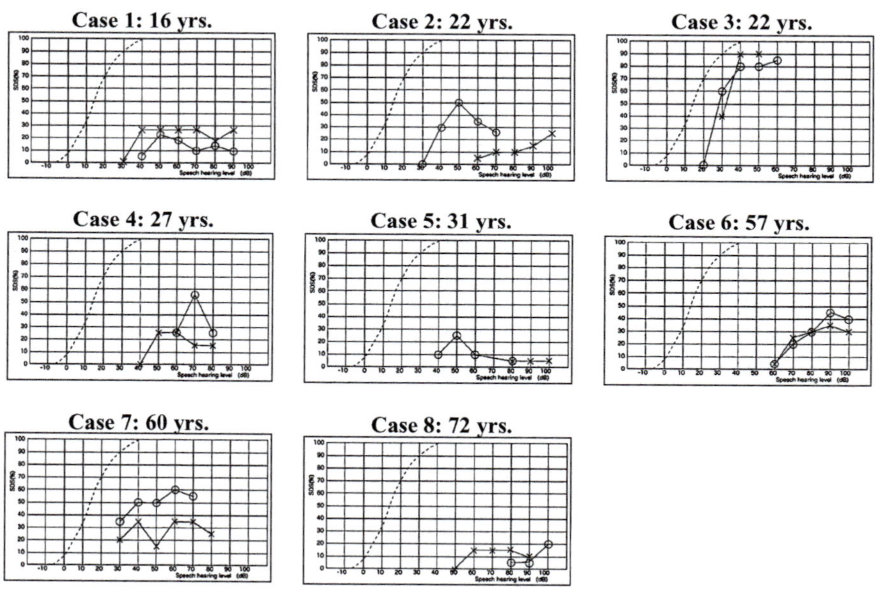

Fig. 3. Speech audiograms. The maximum speech discrimination using monosyllables in all patients is below 50%, except in patient 3

Case No.	1	2	3	4	5	6	7	8
DPOAE	+	+	+	+	+	+	+	+
EcochG	-SP	-SP	-SP	-SP	-SP	-SP	-SP	-SP
ABR	–	–	–	–	–	–	–	–

Fig. 4. Summary of objective audiometry of eight patients. *SP*, summating potential

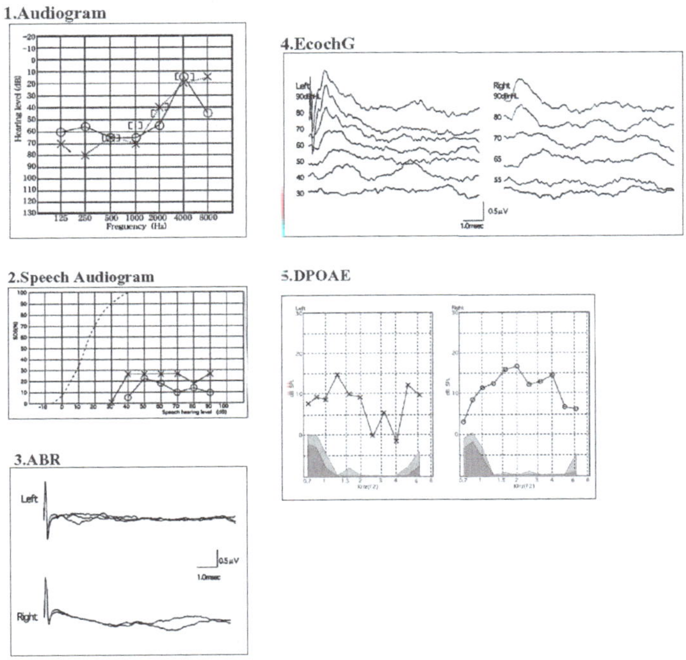

Fig. 5. Case 1: five auditory tests results

Vestibular Assessment Results

Neurologically, motor system evaluation was normal in all patients, except in a 31-year-old woman. Mann test showed abnormal results with eyes closed in five patients. Caloric stimulation with 2 ml ice water provoked normal horizontal nystagmus only in three patients but abnormal responses in the other five patients. In five patients, the VEMP was abolished but in one patient the VEMP was well elicited only in the left (Fig. 6). Vestibular tests recordings of case 3 (Fig. 7), and case 7 (Fig. 8) are shown.

Fig. 6. Case 6: normal caloric reaction and normal vestibular-evoked myogenic potentials (VEMP)

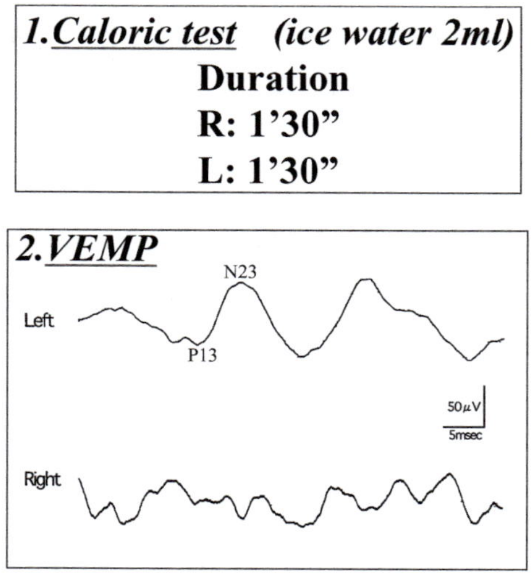

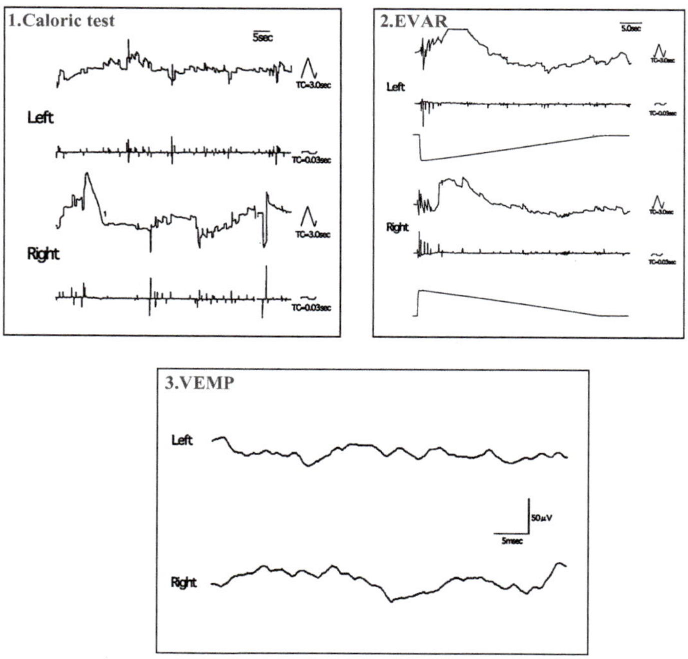

Fig. 7. Case 3: loss of caloric reaction and VEMP

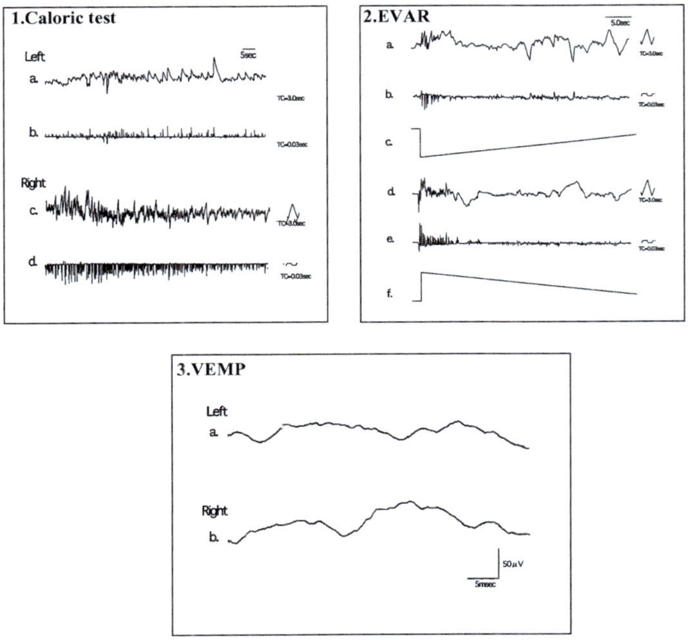

Fig. 8. Case 7: normal caloric reaction and damped rotation (EVAR) but loss of VEMP

Discussion

Our five AN patients each had simultaneous hearing and balance problems, and their complaints have not changed over the past few years. Clinical tests of the balance system in these patients indicated abnormality on the Mann test with eyes closed. Ice water caloric stimulation failed to elicit nystagmus in these patients. Strong rotational testing gave results consistent with bilaterally impaired function of the horizontal semicircular canals and/or vestibular nerves.

In the same five patients, the VEMP was abolished. The VEMP apparently disappears after a unilateral vestibular nerve section with preservation of hearing and is probably of saccular origin. Absence of the VEMP is probably the result of the pathology of the inferior vestibular nerve or the sacculus. However, the other three patients did not show vestibular abnormality.

We suggest the use of the term "auditory neuropathy only" and "auditory-vestibular neuropathy" [3,4] and "vestibular neuropathy only" [5] in AN to characterize these patients with involvement of only the auditory branch of the VIII cranial nerve, both the auditory and vestibular branch. This terminology may help to categorize this disorder more pathophysiologically.

In conclusion, auditory nerve disease should be classified into three types by the presence or absence of involvement of the vestibular nerve pathophysiologically in addition to the auditory nerve. In our study, it is emphasized that there is auditory neuropathy only, and auditory and vestibular pathology and vestibular neuropathy only.

Acknowledgments This work was supported by a Grant for Research on Sensory and Communicative Disorders (H18-Kankakuki-general-003) from the Ministry of Health, Labour and Welfare, and by a Grant-in-Aid for Scientific Research from Areas (A)(2)-15209055 from the Ministry of Education, Culture, Sports Science and Technology of Japan.

References

1. Kaga K, Nakamura M, Shinogami M, et al (1996) Auditory nerve disease of both ears revealed by auditory brainstem responses, electrocochleography, and otoacoustic emission. Scand Audiol 25:233–238
2. Starr A, Picton TW, Sininger Y, et al (1996) Auditory neuropathy. Brain 119:741–753
3. Kaga K, Iwasaki S, Tamura A, et al (1997) Temporal bone pathology of acoustic neuroma correlating with presence of electrocochleography and absence of auditory brainstem response. J Laryng Otol 111:967–972
4. Sheykholeslami K, Kaga K, Kaga M (2001) An isolated and sporadic auditory neuropathy (auditory nerve disease): report of five patients. J Laryngol Otol 115:530–534
5. Baloh RW, Jacobson K, Honrubia V (1989) Idiopathic bilateral vestibulopathy. Neurology 39:272–275

Identification of Different Subtypes of Auditory Neuropathy Using Electrocochleography

Catherine M. McMahon[1], Robert B. Patuzzi[2], William P.R. Gibson[3], and Halit Sanli[4]

Summary

Currently, the physiological mechanisms underlying auditory neuropathy are unclear, and there are likely to be multiple sites of lesion. A better understanding of the disruption in individual cases may lead to more effective management and device selection. Frequency-specific round-window electrocochleography (ECochG) waveforms were used to assess local hair cell, dendritic, and axonal currents generated within the cochlea in 15 subjects with auditory neuropathy (16 ears). These results were compared with electrically evoked auditory brainstem response (EABR) measured after cochlear implantation. The results of this study demonstrate that predominantly two patterns of ECochG waveforms can be identified: (i) a prolonged latency of the hair cell summating potential (SP) waveform with or without residual CAP activity and (ii) a normal latency SP, typically followed by a dendritic potential (DP). We show that seven of eight subjects with a prolonged SP showed a normal EABR waveform, consistent with a presynaptic lesion, whereas six of seven subjects with a normal latency SP showed poor morphology or absent EABR waveforms, consistent with a postsynaptic lesion. We suggest that a presynaptic and postsynaptic type of auditory neuropathy exist, which may have implications for the fitting of cochlear implants.

Key words Auditory neuropathy, Electrocochleography, Cochlear microphonic, Summating potential, Cochlear implantation

Introduction

Auditory neuropathy (AN) is classified by normal cochlear mechanical function, shown by present otoacoustic emissions (OAEs) and/or cochlear microphonic

[1]Centre for Language Sciences, Macquarie University, Syndey, NSW 2109, Australia

[2]Department of Physiology, School of Biomedical and Chemical Sciences, University of Western Australia, Perth, WA, Australia

[3]Department of Surgery, University of Sydney, Sydney, NSW, Australia

[4]Sydney Cochlear Implant Centre, Sydney, NSW, Australia

doi: 10.1007/978-4-431-09433-3_3,

waveforms, but absent or severely disrupted synchronous neural activity, observed as an absent or grossly abnormal auditory brainstem response (ABR) waveform [1]. A consequence of this broad classification is that AN may encompass multiple sites of lesion, including disruption to inner hair cells, the primary afferent synapse, or the auditory brainstem [1,2]. It is likely that this accounts for at least some of the variability in the functional outcomes of hearing aid fitting or cochlear implantation reported previously [3–5]. Therefore, more accurate classification of AN into specific sites of lesion is needed. Scalp recording techniques, typically used for ABR measurements, have shown variable amounts of cochlear activity [6]. However, round-window electrocochleography (ECochG) provides a higher-quality recording of basally located hair cell and dendritic currents, which are in closer proximity to the recording electrode [7,8]; this is important in the differential diagnosis of cochlear disruptions, such as AN, where the generation of action potentials relies on a cascade of events. That is, vibration of the basilar membrane, which is enhanced by outer hair cell (OHC) activity, causes depolarisation of inner hair cells (IHCs), which leads to transmitter release and the generation of excitatory postsynaptic currents, ultimately initiating action potentials. The extracellular potentials that are generated by these events, and can be measured from the round window, include the cochlear microphonic (CM), the summating potential (SP), the dendritic potential (DP), and the compound action potential (CAP). The CM is an alternating current potential that is dominated by OHC activity (Fig. 1A) [8,9], whereas the SP is a direct current response that arises from the summed response of inner and outer hair cell activity[1] (Fig. 1B) [9]. When measured from the round window using a low-frequency tone, the CM reflects the activity from the basal OHCs [8]. Consistent with this, intracellular recording of the basal OHCs during low-frequency pure tone stimulation in anaesthetised guinea pigs shows a sinusoidal and essentially symmetrical receptor potential [10]. Therefore, a stimulus of alternating polarity should null OHC contributions so that the extracellular SP is dominated by IHC currents (although a smaller contribution from OHCs may remain; Fig. 1B) [11,12]. The broad negative DP, first described by Dolan and colleagues [13], is assumed to be the extracellular correlate of the excitatory postsynaptic currents that precede action potential initiation (Fig. 1C) [14], whereas the CAP represents the synchronous activity of primary afferent neurons (Fig. 1D) [15,16].

The present study is a retrospective study that aims to investigate the possible physiological mechanisms underlying AN. Sound-evoked ECochG waveforms, obtained using frequency-specific tone-bursts in 15 subjects, are compared with electrically evoked auditory brainstem response (EABR) waveforms obtained during the cochlear implantation surgery (16 ears). In this study, subjects were identified as having AN on the basis of absent sound-evoked ABR waveforms but large click- and tone-burst-evoked CM waveforms (observed in both scalp and round-window recordings). Pure tone hearing thresholds were typically severe to

---

[1]As shown by Sellick et al [14], the SP waveform may include neural contributions. However, we have assumed that there are no neural contributions to onset of the SP.

profound as almost all these subjects were identified as cochlear implant candidates based on poor behavioral thresholds. The results of this study demonstrate that predominantly two patterns of ECochG waveforms were identified in subjects with AN: (a) an SP (with or without residual neural activity) with a prolonged onset latency, consistent with a disruption of transmitter release or α–amino-3-hydroxy-5-methyl-4-isoxazolepropionic acid (AMPA) channel activation; and (b) a normal onset latency SP followed by DP in most subjects, indicating a failure of spike initiation. We show that there is a correlation between the type of ECochG waveform assessed before implantation and the outcome of cochlear implantation, assessed using EABR. That is, in seven of the eight ears that show a prolonged SP onset latency but no obvious DP, the EABR waveform showed normal waveform morphology, indicating a presynaptic site of lesion. Only one subject showed an absent EABR waveform. However, in six subjects who show a normal latency SP waveform followed by a broad DP, the EABR waveforms were absent (two of seven ears)

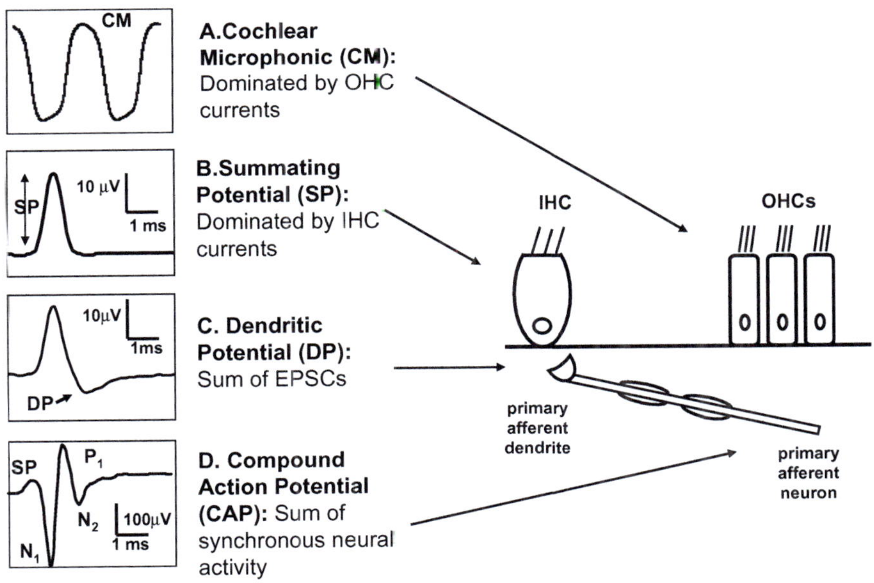

Fig. 1. Four electrocochleography (ECochG) waveforms can be measured from the round window of anaesthetised guinea pig under various conditions (see Sellick et al. 2003 [14]). **A** The cochlear microphonic (*CM*), produced by a single-polarity low-frequency tone, originates from cochlear outer hair cells (*OHCs*). Using an alternating high-frequency tone-burst, the following potentials can be measured. **B** A summating potential (*SP*), dominated by inner hair cell (*IHC*) activity, is shown here after application of kainate to the cochlear round window (which blocks the generation of excitatory postsynaptic potentials). **C** A dendritic potential (*DP*), the sum of excitatory postsynaptic currents (*EPSCs*), is only observed after abolishing spike activity with round-window application of tetrodotoxin. **D** A compound action potential (*CAP*), the synchronous activity from the primary afferent neurons, was measured before application of either kainate or tetrodotoxin

or showed extremely poor morphology (5/7 ears), consistent with a postsynaptic disruption. In these cases, we suggest that the mechanism is likely to arise from either a disruption of the nerve per se, or a disruption of the auditory brainstem.

Materials and Methods

Characteristics of Auditory Neuropathy Subjects

All subjects (9 male, 6 female) were diagnosed with AN between 3 and 24 months of age on the basis of the large CM waveforms, most obvious when produced by lower-frequency single-polarity stimuli during ECochG (Fig. 2B) or ABR (Fig. 2C) measurement, and the absence of the ABR (including waves I and II) using alternating stimuli (Fig. 2D). The CM waveform obtained in most subjects was very similar to the stimulus waveform and was differentiated from the stimulus artifact by the amplitude of the response (at least three times larger than subjects with a profound sensorineural hearing loss, which we assumed was only artifact).

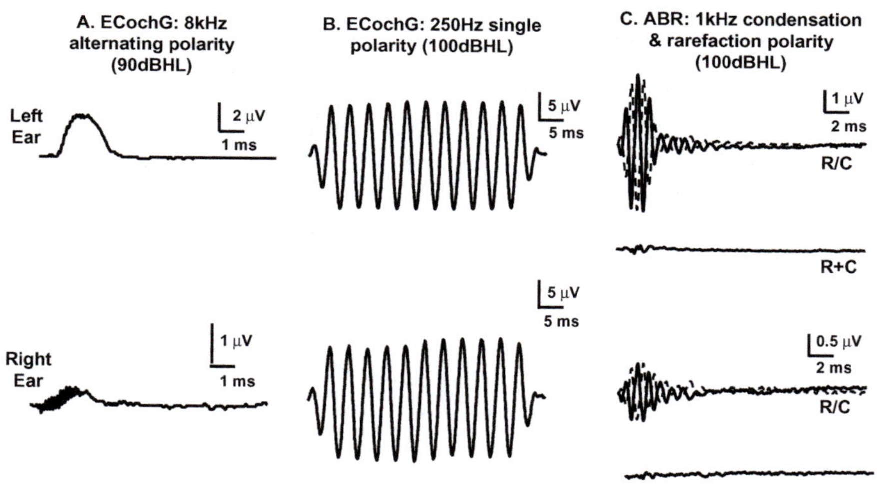

Fig. 2. Electrocochleography (*ECochG*) and auditory brainstem response (*ABR*) waveforms measured in one auditory neuropathy (AN) subject (AN 15) from left (*upper traces*) and right (*lower traces*) ears. **A** ECochG waveforms, produced by an alternating 8-kHz tone-burst (shown here at 90 dB HL), shows a positive summating potential (SP). Incomplete cancellation of the cochlear microphonics can be observed on the SP waveform on the right ear. **B** A symmetrical cochlear microphonic (CM) waveform can be observed using a longer-duration single-polarity low-frequency tone (shown here at 100 dB HL for 50 ms). **C** Auditory brainstem responses measured with single-polarity (R/C) 1-kHz tone-bursts showed large CM waveforms. When these responses were added (R + C) to null the CM, the ABR was absent

All AN subjects showed hearing thresholds in the severe to profound range, except AN 9, who had a moderate to severe loss; this is not the most common finding in AN [17] yet remains one of the criteria for cochlear implant candidacy at the Sydney Cochlear Implant Centre. None of our subjects has shown evidence of additional peripheral neuropathies nor were there any abnormalities observed using magnetic resonance imaging (MRI) or computed tomography (CT) scanning. Many of the AN subjects presented with a medical history of neonatal problems, including prematurity, jaundice, and other complications. However, there were no complications with the pregnancy and birth for approximately half these subjects. There was a possible genetic link in six subjects, five who had siblings also diagnosed with AN, and one with two first cousins with AN. Cochlear implants were fitted between 4 and 53 months after a hearing aid trial and were mostly fitted monaurally (eight left and seven right), with one subject having been fitted bilaterally (Table 1).

Surgical Procedures and Measurement Techniques in Humans

Surgical procedures rarely lasted more than 2 h, and recordings of sound-evoked and electrically evoked round-window ECochG and ABR were made during this time. Access to the round-window niche was made via a posterior myringotomy, and in cases in which otitis media with effusion was present, the serous fluid was aspirated and a ventilation tube inserted. Positioning of the electrode in the RW niche was achieved by eye, visualised through the operating microscope, and secured by a cushioned monaural headset magnetically coupled to a TDH-39 earphone (Telephonics Corp., Farmingdale, NY, USA). Most often, "golf-club" electrodes were used so that the electrode could be positioned on the round-window membrane, minimizing the possibility of membrane damage. However, in cases where the round-window niche could not be easily visualised, straight electrodes were positioned as close to the niche as possible. Electrodes were custom-made from Teflon-coated stainless steel wire stripped bare at the tip, and golf-club electrodes were slightly bent approximately 1 mm from the tip to create the "golf club." An indifferent needle electrode was inserted into the ipsilateral earlobe, and a scalp electrode was sealed onto the vertex of the scalp for later ABR measurements. Over the period of data collection in this study, two different data acquisition systems were used (initially the Medelec Sensor, and later the Medelec Synergy, software version 4; Surrey, UK). There were no differences in the presentation of sound stimuli or data acquisition between these systems. Sound stimuli were presented via the TDH-39 headphone (described above) and included monophasic clicks (0.1 ms in duration) and tone-bursts between 500 Hz to 8 kHz with rise-fall times dependent upon the frequency and a repetition rate of 15/s. To cancel CM activity, the polarity of the stimuli was reversed (i.e., condensation to rarefaction) once (approximately) half the waveform samples were averaged. However, this method resulted in incomplete cancellation of CM waveforms. This incomplete

Table 1. Characteristics of subjects diagnosed with auditory neuropathy (AN) in this study

	Sex	Gestation age (weeks)	Etiology	Diagnosis (months)	Audiometric thresholds	Hearing aid (HA) age (months)	Implantation age (months)	Implant ear
AN1	M	39	Genetic (sibling is AN2)	3	Profound	3	7	R
AN2	F	40	Genetic (sibling is AN1)	3	Profound	3	13	L
AN3	M	40	Genetic (cousin of subjects AN1 and AN2)	3	Profound	4	18	L
AN4	M	41	Induced at 41 weeks, heart rate slowed	3	Severe-profound	10	15	L
AN5	M	40	No medical history	24	Severe-profound	26	69	R
AN6	M	34	Twin, mild jaundice	14	Profound	16	30	R
AN7	M	40	Intrauterine rubella	3	Profound	4	12	R
AN8	F	40	CMV	5	Severe-profound	5	58 (R)/27(L)	R & L
AN9	M	40	Genetic (sibling is AN10)	6	Moderate-severe	9	31	L
AN10	F	40	Genetic (sibling is AN9)	19	Profound	21	64	R
AN11	F	40	Intrauterine CMV, neonatal jaundice	6	Profound	15	36	R
AN12	F	25	Premature, jaundice, hydrocephalus	18	Severe-profound	18	57	L
AN13	M	40	Genetic, Usher's syndrome type 1, developmental delay	23	Profound	31	42	R
AN14	F	40	No medical history	17	Profound	25	31	L
AN15	F	24	Premature	6	Severe-profound	20	40	L

cancellation was most often caused by the asymmetrical distortion in the CM waveform, so that only the fundamental component was cancelled and any remaining oscillatory activity was generally a harmonic of the stimulus frequency. Electrocochleographic responses were sampled over a 10- to 20-ms window, bandpass filtered between 10 Hz and 3 kHz, and amplified according to their relative amplitude (between 2 and 10 μV/division). The number of samples taken for a single average was solely dependent upon the clarity of the trace, but was generally either 128 or 256 samples. Sound-evoked ABR measurements were made using a vertex-ipsilateral earlobe montage. Click stimuli were used to obtain ABR recordings. Averaged ABR waveforms (n = 512 or 1024) were amplified to 0.5 μV/division and bandpass filtered between 100 Hz and 3 kHz.

All subjects included in this study had full insertion of all 22 electrodes of the Nucleus cochlear implant. EABR waveforms were obtained immediately after implantation and using two stimulation modes: monopolar (MP1 + 2) and/or bipolar (BP + 2) at a stimulation rate of 31 pps. A current level of 228 implant units with a pulse width of 25 μs was used in all MP1 + 2 recordings and 100 μs in BP + 2 recordings. Waveforms that appeared poor using this stimulus paradigm were assessed further using increasing pulse widths (25, 37, 50, 75, and 100 μs) and current levels (228, 236, 244, 252). The highest levels of current that were reached were for MP 1 + 2 and were 100 μs at a current level of 252. Levels beyond this were not assessed. Classification of the EABR waveforms into each category (present, absent, or poor waveform morphology) were based on wave V of the EABR. This classification was conducted by two independent clinical audiologists and was primarily based on the waveforms obtained for BP + 2 modes of stimulation. However, where the waveform was not absent, then the highest current levels used for BP + 2 were compared to that obtained for MP1 + 2.

Results

Round-Window Electrocochleography Waveforms

Round-window ECochG waveforms in AN subjects were elicited by brief duration tone-bursts at octave frequencies from 250 Hz to 8 kHz and, in some cases, a longer duration (50-ms) tone-burst at 250 Hz to clearly show the CM waveform. We have assumed that 8 kHz represents the best frequency of the round window [18], and can therefore be used to demonstrate the presence (or absence) of local hair cell, dendritic, and gross spike activity in the average waveform. An example from one subject (AN 15) is shown in Fig. 2 for left (upper traces) and right (lower traces) ears. The response produced by an 8-kHz tone-burst (Fig. 2A) is typically dominated by a large positive SP waveform. Using a low-frequency 250-Hz tone-burst of longer duration (Fig. 2B), it is evident that the CM was largely symmetrical in these AN subjects. Therefore, we have assumed that the hair cell SP produced by high-frequency tone-bursts and measured from the round window in these subjects was dominated by IHC currents [11,19]. In all AN subjects, click-evoked and tone-burst-evoked ABR waveforms showed reversing CM waveforms with single-polarity waveforms (Fig. 2C, R/C) but were absent when rarefaction and condensation traces were summed (Fig. 2C, R + C). This result was observed as either a flat line or, in some cases, a small positive potential, which is assumed to be the IHC SP (consistent with the SP latency, also reported by Starr et al. 2001 [6]).

Round-window ECochG waveforms produced by an alternating 8-kHz tone-burst and measured from the round window in both ears of 15 AN subjects in this study (i.e., 30 ears) could be described by one of three typical responses: (i) a delayed SP waveform with or without residual CAP activity, observed in 15 ears (Fig. 3A); (ii) a normal latency SP waveform followed by a broad negative DP, observed in 13 ears (Fig. 3B); or (iii) a flat line, observed in 2 ears (not shown). The rapid oscillations superimposed over the SP waveforms (observed in most cases) result from the incomplete cancellation of the CM, most obvious at higher sound levels. The DP was first identified in 1989 although it has not yet been well characterised [13,14,16]. Nonetheless, we have identified the DP in this study by the lack of an increase in latency with a reduction in sound level (in fact the latency of the peak appears shorter); this opposes the *increase* in the latency of the N1 peak of the CAP, observed in normally hearing subjects [15] (shown in Fig. 3C).[2]

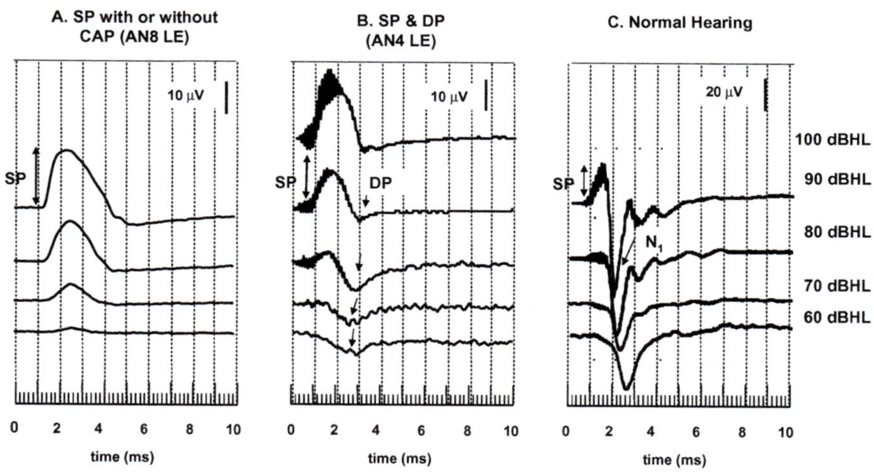

Fig. 3. Examples of the two different types of electrocochleography waveforms in AN subjects (**A**, **B**) compared with a normally hearing subject (**C**). Waveforms were measured with an alternating polarity 8-kHz tone-burst at various sound levels (shown here from 60 to 100 dB HL) show a delayed summating potential (SP) waveform (with or without a residual CAP) (**A**) or a normal latency summating potential (SP) waveform followed by a broad negative dendritic potential (DP) waveform (**B**). Note that the DP latency (**B**) does not increase with decreasing sound level, unlike the N1 of the CAP (**C**)

[2]It was reported by Dolan et al. [13] that the latency of the DP shifted with increasing sound level. However, we have not observed this in our laboratory during measurement of the DP from the RW of anaesthetised guinea pigs (data not shown).

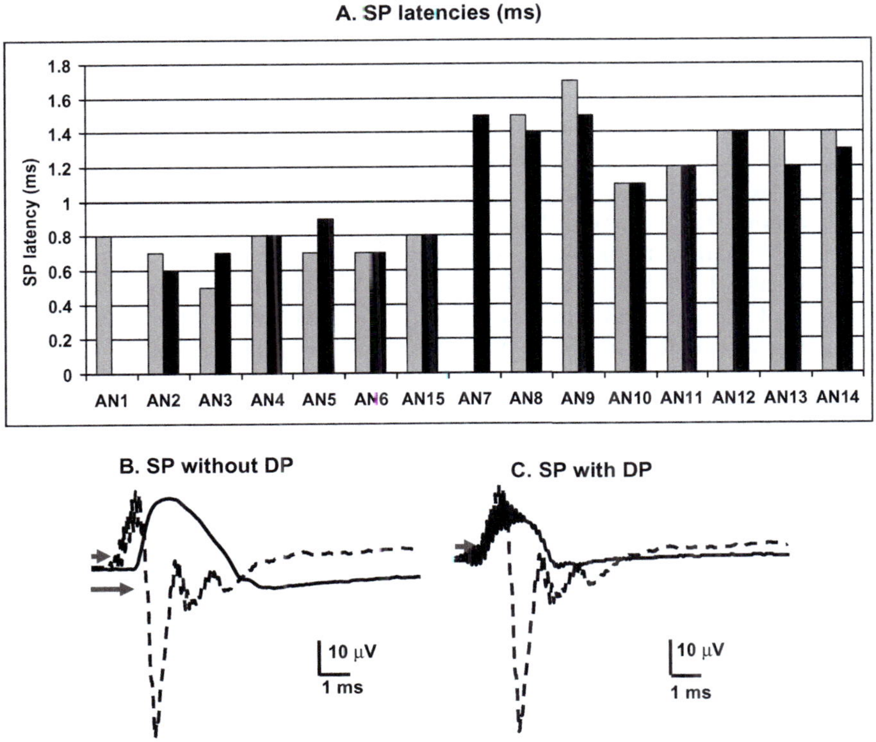

Fig. 4. **A** Comparison of the onset latency of the SP waveform in all 15 AN subjects (left and right ears) without (**B**) and with (**C**) a DP waveform. This finding demonstrates that the SP latency is prolonged in all subjects with no obvious DP but within normal limits in those with a clear DP waveform

Latency of SP Waveforms

The latency of the onset of the SP waveform was measured for all subjects in this study (Fig. 4). Although the sound level used to elicit the SP waveform varied (due to the retrospective nature of this study), we have measured this for sound levels at 90 dB HL, where possible. In any case, the latency of the SP waveform does not significantly change at high sound levels (see Fig. 3 for an example). In 15 ears where there was no obvious DP (AN 7–14; Fig. 4B), the latency of the SP waveform was significantly delayed (>1.0 ms), where the mean latency was 1.35 ms (±0.17 ms), whereas in those 13 subjects where the DP was present (AN 1–6 and AN 15; Fig. 4C), the mean latency of the SP was 0.73 ms (±0.10 ms). Separation of the ECochG responses into these two subgroups showed a significant difference in latency of the SP (using Student's *t* test where $P < 0.01$).

Comparison of ECochG with Implanted EABR

Of the 15 AN subjects at the time of this study, 14 had received monaural cochlear implants (5 right and 8 left) and 1 had sequential bilateral implants. The outcomes of cochlear implantation were assessed using EABR immediately after implantation and were compared with the ECochG waveforms observed before cochlear implantation. Three types of EABR were observed, which were typically consistent for all 22 electrodes: a normal EABR waveform (Fig. 5A, right column, shown here for subject AN 8, LE), showing waves II–V (wave I could not be visualised because of the electrical stimulus artifact); an EABR waveform showing poor waveform morphology for wave V (not shown); or an absent EABR waveform

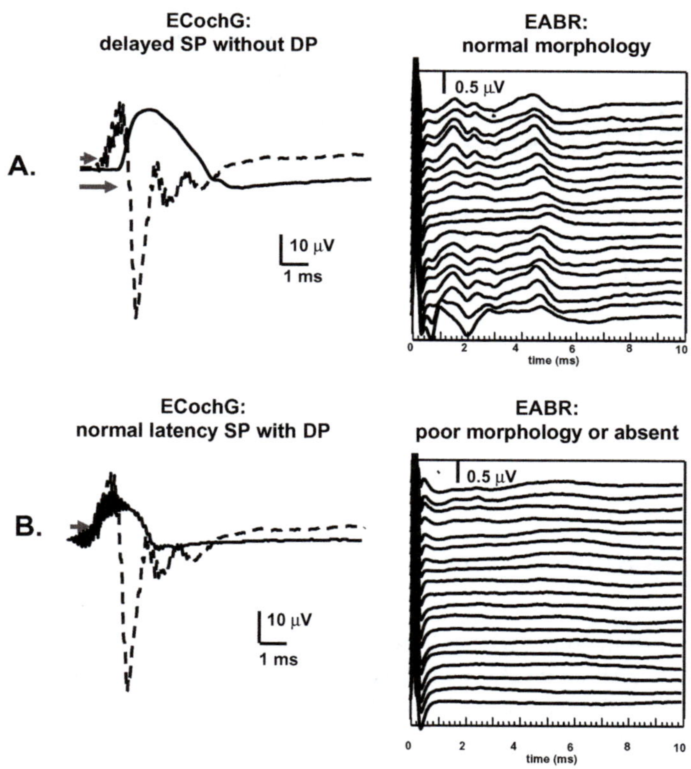

Fig. 5. Correlation between the ECochG waveforms measured before cochlear implantation and electrically evoked ABR (EABR) waveforms observed after cochlear implantation in AN subjects (waveforms shown here were elicited using BP + 2 stimulation mode with a current level of 228 units, pulse width of 100 μs, and rate of 31 pps). **A** Seven of eight ears with a prolonged latency SP showed a normal EABR waveform, consistent with a presynaptic site of lesion. **B** Seven of seven ears with a normal latency SP waveform and a DP showed a poor morphology or absent EABR waveform, consistent with a neural or brainstem lesion

(Fig. 5B, right column, shown here for AN 4, LE). Interestingly, this was not the case for AN 15 who showed absent or poor morphology EABR waveforms for electrodes 1–11 and good waveforms for electrodes 12–22. This finding does demonstrate that this classification is not simple. A subsequent study that we are conducting will address this in more detail. Where the waveforms were determined to be absent or show poor morphology, stimulus artifacts obtained during EABR testing were viewed to ensure that these were normal in appearance. Alternatively, objective testing of the electrode array was conducted using a Crystal Integrity Test to investigate whether the outcome was caused by physiological disruption or malfunction of the implant. The results of this study showed a correlation between the types of ECochG waveform measured before cochlear implantation and the EABR waveform measured after implantation (see Table 2 for a summary). That is, in all subjects who showed a SP and DP, the resultant EABR waveform was either absent or showed poor waveform morphology. On the other hand, for seven of eight subjects (eight of nine ears) who showed a prolonged latency SP waveform with or without residual CAP activity, the EABR appeared normal. AN 14 showed a prolonged SP latency but an absent EABR waveform.

Table 2. Outcomes of electrocochleography (ECochG) measured using an 8-kHz tone-burst before cochlear implantation and electrically evoked acoustic brainstem response (EABR) measured after cochlear implantation in each auditory neuropathy (AN) subject

			SP latency		
Subject	ECochG Right	ECochG Left	Right	Left	EABR (ear implanted)
AN1	SP + DP	Flat line	0.8	N/A	Poor morphology (R)
AN2	SP + DP	SP + DP	0.7	0.6	Poor morphology (L)
AN3	SP + DP	SP + DP	0.5	0.7	Poor morphology (L)
AN4	SP + DP	SP + DP	0.8	0.8	Poor morphology (L)
AN5	SP + DP	SP + DP	0.7	0.9	Absent (L)
AN6	SP + DP	SP + DP	0.7	0.7	Poor morphology (R)
AN15	SP only	SP only	0.8	0.8	Absent/poor morphology for 50% of responses (L)
AN7	Flat line	SP + residual CAP	N/A	1.5	Normal (R)
AN8	SP + residual CAP	SP + residual CAP	1.5	1.4	Normal (L & R)
AN9	SP + residual CAP	SP only	1.7	1.5	Normal (L)
AN10	SP + residual CAP	SP only	1.1	1.1	Normal (R)
AN11	SP + residual CAP	SP + residual CAP	1.2	1.2	Normal (R)
AN12	SP + residual CAP	SP + residual CAP	1.4	1.4	Normal (L)
AN13	SP + residual CAP	SP + residual CAP	1.4	1.2	Normal (L)
AN14	SP + residual CAP	SP only	1.4	1.3	Absent (L)

R, right; L, left

ECochG waveforms were described on the basis of the presence or absence of the summating potential (SP), dendritic potential (DP), or residual compound action potential (CAP), and on the onset latency of the SP waveform

The EABR waveforms were described as normal, poor morphology (based on wave V morphology), or absent

Discussion

The results of this study suggest that frequency-specific ECochG measured from the cochlear round window can be used to identify pre- and postsynaptic disruptions in AN subjects. Presynaptic lesions can be identified by the presence of a delayed latency SP waveform (typically observed with a residual CAP), whereas the presence of the normal latency SP and a present broad negative DP can be used to identify postsynaptic lesions. This finding is supported by the electrophysiological outcomes of cochlear implantation where seven of eight subjects who showed a presynaptic site of lesion showed good EABR waveforms assessed after cochlear implantation whereas all seven subjects identified with a postsynaptic disruption showed poor morphology or absent EABR waveforms after cochlear implantation.

Although the results of this study indicate that ECochG is a useful tool in the identification of subtypes of AN, there are some limitations. First, the measurement of ECochG in this study was conducted under a general anaesthetic to minimise any potential movement of the child. While this is a valuable tool for assessing thresholds in children who are difficult to test or who do not show any behavioral thresholds, it is not routinely used in clinical practice in young children. Second, the round-window recording provides detailed information about cochlear hair cell and dendritic potentials generated at or near the recording electrode [7,8]. However, as local potentials decay exponentially with distance from the recording electrodes [20], the responses obtained are generated from basal hair cells and dendrites only. Therefore, it must be assumed that the pattern of disruption is similar throughout the cochlear length. Although this is an obvious limitation, in the case of AN where the underlying physiological mechanisms are not clear, we believe that the benefits of this technique outweigh these shortcomings.

Electrophysiological Support for Presynaptic Mechanisms of Auditory Neuropathy

In the seven subjects (eight ears) who showed a delay in the SP onset of the 8-kHz ECochG waveform and normal EABR waveforms, it is assumed that the site of lesion is presynaptic. The round-window SP waveform is composed of contributions from both inner and outer hair cells, although it appears to be dominated by activity from IHCs under normal physiological conditions (see [12] for a review). While it may be possible that some amount of OHC disruption occurs in AN, where OAEs can sometimes disappear over time [21], it is generally accepted that OHC activity is largely preserved in this disorder (shown by the presence of the CM waveform). Therefore, we believe that the delay in the SP waveform shown in this study is the result of changes to IHC activity. Disruption to the otoferlin gene has recently been demonstrated to be a cause of auditory neuropathy in some subjects with profound hearing thresholds [22,23]. In particular, this gene has been found to be necessary for transmitter release at the IHC ribbon synapse [24]. Although this is a potential mechanism of presynaptic AN, disruption of transmitter release per se would not alter the onset latency of the IHC current during sound stimulation and therefore the SP. Therefore, we present an alternative explanation here. Assuming that the round-window SP produced by an 8-kHz tone-burst is dominated by IHC activity in that region, then the delay in the SP latency during the Gaussian tone-bursts used could be produced by static displacement of the operating point (P_0) of the IHC hair bundle. This shift would be oriented towards the closed, saturated part of the IHC transfer curve relating hair bundle angle to IHC current, so that almost all mechanoelectrical transduction (MET) channels exist in the closed state in silence (i.e., a direction consistent with a basilar membrane shift towards scala tympani; Fig. 6A). A shift in the operating point of the IHCs would have a number of implications for the generation of the IHC current, transmitter release, and, subsequently, spike generation. First, the time taken for the channels to move from a closed state into an open state would produce a delay in the onset of the IHC current and, therefore, the latency of the SP waveform. Second, a reduced number of channels in an open state under resting conditions would reduce the standing current through these cells (i.e., the silent current) [25], hyperpolarizing the IHC resting membrane potential. As a result, a greater depolarisation of the IHCs would be required to trigger the vesicular release of neurotransmitter [26]. That is, while increased sound levels are typically required to produce a clear SP

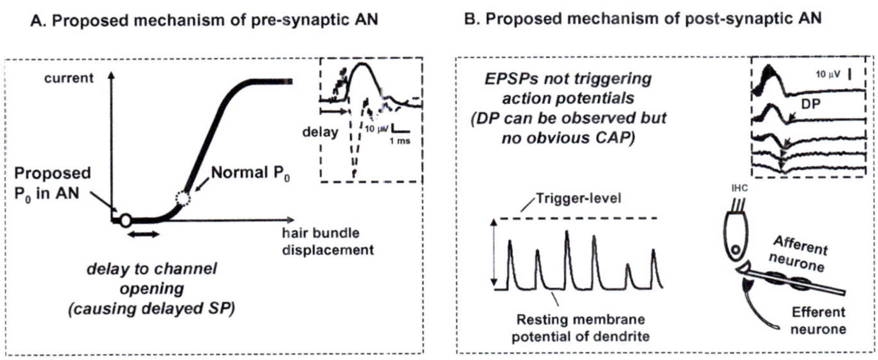

Fig. 6. Proposed mechanisms of presynaptic and postsynaptic AN. **A** Presynaptic auditory neuropathy. The delayed onset latency of the SP could be produced by a static shift in the operating point in a direction toward the scala tympani (ST); this would reduce the number of channels in an open state in silence. As a result, there would be a delay in the opening of the mechanoelectrical transduction (MET) channels and, therefore, a delay in the current through the inner hair cells (IHCs), increasing the SP latency; and hyperpolarisation of the cell so that more current (a greater depolarisation) is required for transmitter to be released for action potential generation, resulting in an increased SP/CAP ratio. **B** Postsynaptic auditory neuropathy. The presence of the DP indicates that EPSPs are being generated but are not triggering an action potential; this may either result from an increase in the voltage needed to trigger an action potential (trigger level) or a decrease in the membrane potential of the dendrite so that the EPSPs cannot reach the critical voltage needed. Alternatively, this could also result from a disruption to the voltage-gated channels that are needed to produce an action potential

waveform, the release of transmitter is reduced, thereby inhibiting excitatory postsynaptic potential (EPSP) generation and spike initiation. This would either reduce the number of EPSPs *and* the number of spikes initiated, resulting in a small CAP waveform, or abolish all EPSP and spike activity, resulting in an absent CAP waveform.

Electrophysiological Support for Postsynaptic Mechanisms of Auditory Neuropathy

Seven subjects showed a normal latency SP followed by a broad negative DP and EABR waveforms that were either absent or showed poor waveform morphology. The DP cannot be observed in normally hearing subjects, where it is assumed to be obscured by the much larger CAP waveform and, of course, the membrane potential approaches the Na^+ equilibrium potential at the top of the intracellular spike, minimizing the Na^+ driving potential and altering the shape of the DP observed in the absence of spike activity. Therefore, the presence of the DP without any additional neural activity (except at higher sound levels) indicates that transmitter release and EPSP generation were essentially normal, but spike initiation was grossly disrupted. Because the latency of the SP was also not altered, we have assumed that the IHC operating point and resting membrane potential were normal in these subjects.

The disruption to the EABR waveform suggests that the site of lesion is possibly at the primary afferent neurones per se or a disruption of the auditory brainstem resulting in cochlear efferent dysfunction. Although it is currently not clear how disruption of the cochlear efferent neurons can lead to a significant disruption of neural synchrony because sectioning of these neurons at the olivocochlear bundle leads to small changes in threshold only [27], the lateral efferent neurons are ideally positioned to affect the success of action potential generation [27,28]. A disruption of the afferent neurons in these subjects may have resulted from a failure of the EPSPs to reach the critical voltage required to activate voltage-gated Na^+ channels and the primary afferent action potential (Fig. 6B) [29,30], either because the primary afferent membrane was hyperpolarised at the site of spike initiation, or because the activation voltage of the Na^+ channels itself was greater than normal. Alternatively, voltage-gated Na^+ channels may have been disrupted or inactivated (consistent with the model proposed previously; see [31]).

Conclusions

In this study, subjects with AN showed presynaptic and postsynaptic sites of disruption. In most cases, the EABR results obtained after cochlear implantation are consistent with this finding. That is, in cases that show a presynaptic lesion,

EABR results were normal whereas in those showing a postsynaptic lesion, EABR results were absent or abnormal. This was not the case for one AN subject who showed ECochG responses consistent with a presynaptic lesion, however; EABR results obtained after cochlear implantation were absent (AN 14). No medical complications were reported for the pregnancy or birth, nor was a genetic component identified. However, it does highlight the possibility that AN may define cases in which where there are more than a single lesion of the peripheral auditory system. It is clear that separation of AN into different sites of lesion may guide more effective clinical decision making about interventions, particularly the use of different hearing devices. Frequency-specific ECochG appears to be the most useful clinical tool to undertake this, providing more detail than scalp measurements of the presence or absence of various cochlear potentials.

References

1. Starr A, Picton T, Sininger Y, et al (1996) Auditory neuropathy. Brain 119:741–753
2. Rance G (2005) Auditory neuropathy/dys-synchrony and its perceptual consequences. Trends Amplif 9:1–43
3. Buss E, Labadie RF, Brown CJ, et al (2002) Outcome of cochlear implantation in pediatric auditory neuropathy. Otol Neurotol 23:328–332
4. Rance G, Cone-Wesson B, Wunderlich J, et al (2002) Speech perception and cortical event related potentials in children with auditory neuropathy. Ear Hear 23:239–253
5. Miyamoto RT, Kirk KI, Renshaw J, et al (1999) Cochlear implantation in auditory neuropathy. Laryngoscope 109:181–185
6. Starr A, Sininger Y, Nguyen T, et al (2001) Cochlear receptor (microphonic and summating potentials, otoacoustic emissions) and auditory pathway (auditory brain stem potentials) activity in auditory neuropathy. Ear Hear 22:91–99
7. Ghiz AF, Salt AN, DeMott JE, et al (2001) Quantitative anatomy of the round window and cochlear aqueduct in guinea pigs. Hear Res 162:105–112
8. Patuzzi RB, Yates GK, Johnstone BM (1989) The origin of the low-frequency microphonic in the first cochlear turn of guinea-pig. Hear Res 39:177–188
9. Dallos P (1973) The auditory periphery: biophysics and physiology. Academic Press, New York
10. Russell IJ, Sellick PM (1983) Low-frequency characteristics of intracellularly recorded receptor potentials in guinea-pig cochlear hair cells. J Physiol 338:179–206
11. Zheng XY, Ding DL, McFadden SL, et al (1997) Evidence that inner hair cells are the major source of cochlear summating potentials. Hear Res 113:76–88
12. Durrant JD, Wang J, Ding DL, et al (1998) Are inner or outer hair cells the source of summating potentials recorded from the round window? J Acoust Soc Am 104:370–376
13. Dolan DF, Xi L, Nuttall AL (1989) Characterization of an EPSP-like potential recorded remotely from the round window. J Acoust Soc Am 86:2167–2171
14. Sellick P, Patuzzi R, Robertson D (2003) Primary afferent and cochlear nucleus contributions to extracellular potentials during tone-bursts. Hear Res 176:42–58
15. Kiang NYS, Watanabe T, Thomas EC, et al (1965) Discharge patterns of single fibres in the cat's auditory nerve. Research Monograph no. 35. MIT Press, Cambridge
16. McMahon CM, Patuzzi RB (2002) The origin of the 900 Hz spectral peak in spontaneous and sound-evoked round-window electrical activity. Hear Res 173:134–152

17. Starr A, Sininger YS, Pratt H (2000) The varieties of auditory neuropathy. J Basic Clin Physiol Pharmacol 11:215–230
18. O'Leary SJ, Mitchell TE, Gibson WP, et al (2000) Abnormal positive potentials in round window electrocochleography. Am J Otol 21:813–818
19. Patuzzi R, Sellick PM (1983) A comparison between basilar membrane and inner hair cell receptor potential input-output functions in the guinea pig cochlea. J Acous Soc Am 74:1734–1741
20. Withnell R (2001) The cochlear microphonic as an indication of outer hair cell function. Ear Hear 22:75–77
21. Deltenre P, Mansbach AL, Bozet C, et al (1999) Auditory neuropathy with preserved cochlear microphonics and secondary loss of otoacoustic emissions. Audiology 38:187–195
22. Rodríguez-Ballesteros M, del Castillo FJ, Martín Y, et al (2003) Auditory neuropathy in patients carrying mutations in the otoferlin gene (OTOF). Hum Mutat 22:451–456
23. Varga R, Kelley PM, Keats BJ, et al (2003) Non-syndromic recessive auditory neuropathy is the result of mutations in the otoferlin (OTOF) gene. J Med Genet 40:45–50
24. Roux I, Safieddine S, Nouvian R, et al (2006) Otoferlin, defective in a human deafness form, is essential for exocytosis at the auditory ribbon synapse. Cell 127:277–289
25. Zidanic M, Brownell WE (1990) Fine structure of the intracochlear potential field. I. The silent current. Biophys J 57:1253–1268
26. Moser T, Beutner D (2000) Kinetics of exocytosis and endocytosis at the cochlear inner hair cell afferent synapse of the mouse. Proc Natl Acad Sci U S A 97:883–888
27. Liberman MC (1990) Effects of chronic cochlear de-efferentation on auditory-nerve response. Hear Res 49:209–223
28. Le Prell CG, Shore SE, Hughes LF, et al (2003) Disruption of lateral efferent pathways: functional changes in auditory evoked responses. J Assoc Res Otolaryngol 4:276–290
29. Katsuki Y, Yanagisawa K, Kanzaki J (1966) Tetraethylammonium and tetrodotoxin: effects on cochlear potentials. Science 151:1544–1545
30. Lin X (1997) Action potentials and underlying voltage-dependent currents studied in cultured spiral ganglion neurons of the postnatal gerbil. Hear Res 108:157–179
31. Schmiedt RA, Okamura HO, Lang H, et al (2002) Ouabain application to the round window of the gerbil cochlea: a model of auditory neuropathy and apoptosis. J Assoc Res Otolaryngol 3:223–233

Sound Localization and Lateralization of Patients with Auditory Neuropathy

Kenji Itoh[1], Sozo Kuroki[1], Sotaro Sekimoto[1], and Kimitaka Kaga[2]

Summary

To investigate the spatial abilities of patients with auditory neuropathy (auditory nerve disease, AN), we applied a sound localization task with a speaker array as well as a binaural sound lateralization task. In the sound localization task, subjects were asked to choose the direction of actual sound source of short (duration, 3 ms) or long (duration, 100 ms) noise bursts centered at 500 Hz played from 1 of 12 surrounding (220°) speakers. The AN patients identified the direction of the long-duration sound fairly well. However, they could localize few sources of the short-duration sound. The results were compared with non-AN patients and normal persons to discuss the auditory neural processing of cues for transient or prolonged source estimation, that is, interaural intensity and time differences (IID, ITD) and spectral difference by head-related transfer function (HRTF).

Key words Sound localization, Head-related transfer function, Binaural interaction, Temporal resolution, Neurosynaptic system

Introduction

In a free sound field, auditory spatial cues are not limited to binaural differences in intensity and/or delay and some monaural or interaural spectral shape cues in elevation and also in azimuth by head-related transfer function (HRTF) [1,2].

To investigate the auditory spatial abilities of patients with auditory neuropathy (ANP) [3,4], we applied a two-dimensional sound localization test with a speaker array as well as the common binaural lateralization test with a headphone.

[1]Department of Sensory and Motor Neuroscience, The University of Tokyo School of Medicine 7-3-1, Hongo, Bunkyo-ku, Tokyo 113-0033, Japan

[2]National Institute of Sensory Organs, National Tokyo Medical Center, 2-5-1 Higashigaoka, Megur-ku, Tokyo 152-8902, Japan

doi: 10.1007/978-4-431-09433-3_4,

The lateralization and localization results on perceived spatial pattern and magnitude of localization errors of ANPs were compared with conductive hearing-impaired persons with some hearing aids as well as normal persons. The individual detectability on lateralization of binaural moving fused images was tested before the localization paradigm.

Material and Methods

Three subjects with auditory neuropathy were selected for the experiments through clinical and audiological tests including examination on sound lateralization by interaural intensity (IID) and interaural time differences (ITD) (Table 1a). Four participants with bilateral conductive hearing loss and seven normal persons were included as controls.

The lateralization of sound image was achieved by the gradual IID change (1 dB/s) under fixed ITD or ITD change (50 μs/s) under fixed IID of narrowband (420–561 Hz) noise bursts. The direction of gradual change was reversed after the subject responded with the left or right button at the detection of movement of the image to the left or right, respectively.

Sound localization testing was performed for each subject in an anechoic chamber served by a horizontal arc array of 12 uniform compact monitor speakers (100PR; Bose, Framingham, MA, USA) spanning 220° with a spacing of 20°. Each monitor speaker was located on a dedicated floor stand at ear level of the subject sitting at the center of the arc with a radius of 2 m (Fig. 1).

The test stimuli for localization in the horizontal plane were the same as the noise burst for the lateralization, but with duration of either 3 ms or 100 ms. The stimulus sounds were generated digitally and delivered to 1 of 12 channels on six stereo power amplifiers (P-60D; TOA, Kobe, Japan) under a custom computer-controlled localization system (RION, Tokyo, Japan). Localization was tested for each short or long stimulus in separate runs. The stimuli were individually adjusted at 40 dB SL through prior threshold tests.

Table 1. Details of subjects and localization results
(a) Clinical and audiological data of subjects with auditory neuropathy (AN)

Subject	AN 1	AN 2	AN 3
Sex/age (years)	F/61	F/67	M/35
L/R pure tone average (dB)	48/43	51/78	95/85
L/R speech score (%)	20/15	10/0	0/0
IID sound lateralization	Detected	Failed	Detected
ITD sound lateralization	Failed	Failed	Failed
L/R OAEs	Normal/normal	Normal/normal	Normal/normal
L/R ABR	Absent/absent	Absent/absent	Absent/absent

AN, auditory neuropathy; F/M, female/male; L/R, left ear/right ear; IID, interaural intensity difference; ITD, interaural time difference; OAEs, otoacoustic emissions; ABR, auditory brainstem response

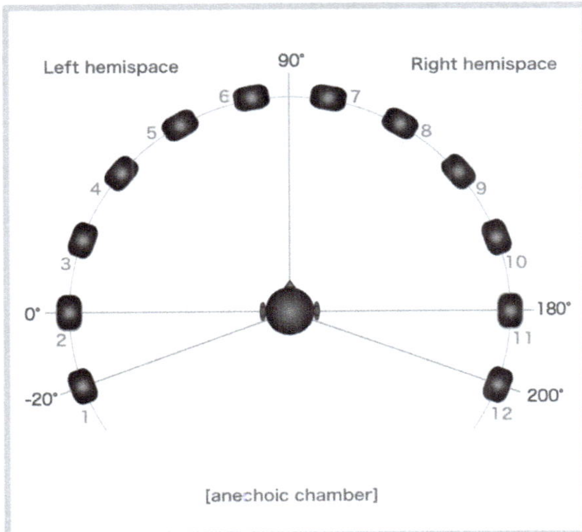

Fig. 1. Speaker array. Twelve speakers were arranged at 20° intervals on a circular arc with radius 3 m in an anechoic chamber. Subjects sat at the center holding a response box

The subject was asked to respond by pushing the corresponding switch in an arc array representing the location of speakers as quickly as possible during a pause of 3 s following each play. In each run, the test stimulus was played three times per sound direction ($3 \times 12 = 36$ trials).

Results

Results on lateralization for AN subjects are given in Table 1a. All AN subjects failed the ITD discrimination test, but two of three subjects showed ability on IID lateralization.

Results on localization for all AN subjects, controls with conductive hearing loss, and normals are given in Table 1b. Overall, AN subjects could barely perform the tasks to localize sounds in a free field. The percentage of responses by AN subjects was less than half in total and less than one-third for the short sound. The non-AN controls both with and without hearing loss answered almost all sounds.

A large discrepancy appeared between hearing loss groups and normals in the accuracy of responding to the direction of the sounds. Normal controls could correctly localize more than 90% of directed sounds within ±20° in the horizontal plane even though there existed a limit on pointing to the exact directions of sounds. Both the hearing loss groups, with and without AN, were unable to localize more than half of either short and long stimuli.

Table 1. Details of subjects and localization results
(b) Group data of sound localization

Group [mean age/*n* (F/M)]	AN [54.3/*n* = 3(2/1)]	Bilateral HI [11.0/*n* = 4(1/3)]	Normal [25.9/*n* = 7(3/4)]
Response (%)			
Total	48.6 ± 18.6	99.0 ± 2.9	98.8 ± 1.8
3 ms NB	31.5 ± 18.2	97.9 ± 4.2	98.4 ± 1.5
100 ms NB	65.7 ± 19.0	100.0 ± 0.0	99.2 ± 2.1
Correct (%)			
3 ms NB	4.6 ± 2.7	13.9 ± 6.0	61.5 ± 10.1
(in response)	(14.7 ± 8.5)	(14.2 ± 6.1)	(62.5 ± 10.2)
100 ms NB	10.2 ± 3.3	14.6 ± 9.5	73.8 ± 12.7
(in response)	(15.5 ± 4.9)	(14.6 ± 9.5)	(74.4 ± 12.8)
Correct ≤ ±20° (%)			
3 ms NB	13.0 ± 7.5	35.4 ± 4.7	94.0 ± 5.2
(in responses)	(41.2 ± 23.8)	(36.1 ± 4.8)	(95.6 ± 5.3)
100 ms NB	28.7 ± 8.9	38.9 ± 9.6	96.4 ± 4.5
(in responses)	(43.7 ± 13.5)	(38.9 ± 9.6)	(97.2 ± 4.5)

HI, conductive hearing-impaired patients with 500 Hz thresholds of 57/63 dB HL (receiving bilateral bone-conduction hearing aids); NB, narrowband (420–561 Hz) noise burst

The spatial patterns of responses and deviated (more than ±40°) answers to short and long stimuli are shown for each group in Fig. 2. Normals responded with no deviated answers with a nearly flat distribution over sound locations. However, the responses with some deviated answers by both AN and non-AN hearing loss groups were remarkably deflected to the left or right side in space for sound direction.

Discussion

The localization test revealed difficulties in sound localization for AN subjects even in sufficient conditions of sound presentation level. Two of three AN subjects complained the sound space within their own head was too small for the external short sounds. Such failures in sound localization by AN subjects may partially caused by the abnormal perceptual distance between sound source and self [5].

The localization patterns in Fig. 2 support the existence of disabilities in detecting the location of sounds. The main cue is confirmed to be ITD for localization of frontal low frequency (<1200 Hz) sounds, including the test stimuli, especially in the horizontal plane [6]. Animal studies indicate that ITD is detected and coded by coincidence neurons in the superior olive complex [7] sending both afferent and efferent outputs for following spatial information processing [8]. The coincidence neurons acquire binaural inputs with precise timing and descent due to neuronal plasticity under a binaurally imbalanced condition [9]. The results from hearing loss groups including subjects with giant magnetostriction bone conduction aids suggest necessary parameters on qualities in time domain and periods of using a hearing aid are necessary for reading clinical localization data [10,11].

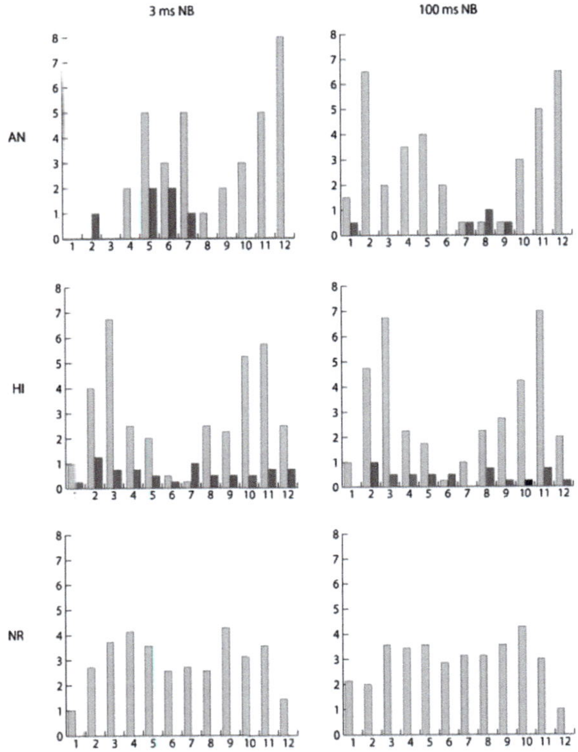

Fig. 2. Performances of normal persons and patients with hearing loss for sound localization. *Light bars*, number of responses per speaker; *dark bars*, number of erratic answers per speaker. *AN*, auditory neuropathy; *HI*, conductive hearing impaired; *NR*, normals

The AN subjects showed a disadvantage, especially in temporal information processing, including speech word recognition, as indicated in recent studies [12]. The initiation data of auditory inputs are important for maintaining good temporal resolution and neural group delays [13,14]. Neuronal factors have been proposed to cause variability in auditory electrical responses from AN subjects [15]. Major factors are concentrated on the junction between inner hair cell and auditory nerve ending [16,17] as well as on auditory nerve degeneration [18,19]. However, secondary afferent and efferent plasticity should be considered for explaining both behavioral [20] and neurophysiological abnormalities [21,22].

References

1. Butler RA, Humanski RA, Musicant AD (1990) Binaural and monaural localization of sound in two-dimensional space. Perception 19:241–256
2. Palomäki KJ, Tiitinen H, Mäkinen V, May PJ, Alku P (2005) Spatial processing in human auditory cortex: the effects of 3D, ITD, and ILD stimulation techniques. Cogn Brain Res 24:7640–7647

3. Kaga K, Nakamura M, Shinogami M, et al (1996) Auditory nerve disease of both ears revealed by auditory brainstem responses, electrocochleography and otoacoustic emissions. Scand Audiol 25:233–238
4. Starr A, Picton TW, Sininger Y, et al (1996) Auditory neuropathy. Brain 119:741–753
5. Kulkarni A, Colburn HS (1998) Role of spectral detail in sound-source. Nature (Lond) 396:747–749
6. Shackleton TM, Bowsher JM, Meddis R (1991) Lateralization of very-short-duration tone pulses of low and high frequencies. Q J Exp Psychol A 43:503–516
7. Itoh K (1985) A neuro-synaptic model of auditory-masking and unmasking process. Biol Cybern 52:229–235
8. Joris P, Yin TC (2007) A matter of time: internal delays in binaural processing. Trends Neurosci 30:70–78
9. Darrow KN, Maison SF, Liberman MC (2006) Cochlear efferent feedback balances interaural sensitivity. Nat Neurosci 9:1474–1476
10. Shepherd RK, Roberts LA, Paolini AG (2004) Long-term sensorineural hearing loss induces functional changes in the rat auditory nerve. Eur J Neurosci 20:3131–3140
11. van Hoesel R, Böhm M, Pesch J, et al (2008) Binaural speech unmasking and localization in noise with bilateral cochlear implants using envelope and fine-timing based strategies. J Acoust Soc Am 123:2249–2263
12. Narne VK, Vanaja CS (2008) Speech identification and cortical potentials individuals with auditory neuropathy. Behav Brain Funct 4:15
13. Moore BC (2002) Interference effects and phase sensitivity in hearing. Philos Transact A Math Phys Eng Sci 360:833–858
14. Dreyer A, Delgutte B (2006) Phase locking of auditory-nerve fibers to the envelopes of high-frequency sounds: implications for sound localization. J Neurophysiol 96:2327–2341
15. Santarelli R, Starr A, Michalewski HJ, et al (2008) Neural and receptor cochlear potentials obtained by transtympanic electrocochleography auditory neuropathy. Clin Neurophysiol 119:653–661
16. Moser T, Neef A, Khimich D (2006) Mechanisms underlying the temporal precision of sound coding at the inner hair cell ribbon synapse. J Physiol 576:55–62
17. Roux I, Safieddine S, Nouvian R, et al (2006) Otoferlin, defective in a human deafness form, is essential for exocytosis at the auditory ribbon synapse. Cell 127:277–289
18. Heil P, Neubauer H, Irvine DR, et al (2007) Spontaneous activity of auditory-nerve fibers: insights into stochastic processes at ribbon synapses. J Neurosci 27:8457–8474
19. Ceranic B, Luxon LM (2004) Progressive auditory neuropathy in patients with Leber's hereditary optic neuropathy. J Neurol Neurosurg Psychiatry 75:626–630
20. Aytekin M, Moss CF, Simon JZ (2008) A sensorimotor approach to sound localization. Neural Comput 20:603–635
21. Niu X, Tahera Y, Canlon B (2007) Environmental enrichment to sound activates dopaminergic pathways in the auditory system. Physiol Behav 92:34–39
22. Kral A, Eggermont JJ (2007) What's to lose and what's to learn: development under auditory deprivation, cochlear implants and limits of cortical plasticity. Brain Res Rev 56:259–269

Trends in Genetic Research on Auditory Neuropathy

Tatsuo Matsunaga

Summary

Various etiologies of auditory neuropathy (AN) have been reported, including genetic causes. Genes such as *OTOF* and *pejvakin* cause AN without other associated symptoms, that is, nonsyndromic auditory neuropathy. Syndromic AN, in which AN is associated with other related symptoms, has been frequently reported in hereditary neurological disorders such as Charcot–Marie–Tooth disease and mitochondrial disease. In these neurological disorders, specific genes and mutations that are related to AN are being revealed. AN may be caused by dysfunction of synapses in inner hair cells. For an example, function of inner hair cells is impaired but that of spiral ganglion cells is maintained in knockout mice of the *OTOF* gene. This finding implies that surgery for cochlear implants may be indicated in patients with AN caused by *OTOF* gene mutations because the spiral ganglion cells are preserved.

Key words Auditory neuropathy, Cochlea, Spiral ganglion, Hereditary hearing loss, Genetic test

History of Genetic Research on Auditory Neuropathy

Auditory neuropathy (AN) is a novel clinical concept of auditory disorder that is distinguished from general sensorineural hearing loss and is characterized by audiological test results indicating normal function of outer hair cells and impairment of auditory neurons [1,2]. Various causes have been reported for AN. In approximately half of AN patients, hearing loss is syndromic as a part of symptoms associated with known causes such as hyperbilirubinemia, anoxia, viral infection, high

Laboratory of Auditory Disorders, National Institute of Sensory Organs, National Tokyo Medical Center, 2-5-1 Higashigaoka, Meguro-ku, Tokyo 152-8902, Japan

doi: 10.1007/978-4-431-09433-3_5, © Springer 2009

Table 1. Genetic causes related to nonsyndromic auditory neuropathy (AN)

Autosomal recessive	*OTOF*
	Pejvakin
	GJB2
Autosomal dominant	AUNA1 locus (13q14–21)
X related	AUNX1 locus (Xq23–27.3)
Mitochondrial	T1095C in12S ribosomal RNA

fever, hereditary neurological disorders, and immunological disorders [3]. In the other half, hearing loss is nonsyndromic, that is, the symptom is isolated. In some of the latter patients, autosomal recessive inheritance has been noted. Recently, *OTOF* gene mutations were found as the cause of such autosomal recessive nonsyndromic AN [4]. Then, various mutations, genes, or loci such as the *pejvakin* gene [5], *GJB2* gene, T1095C mutation in mitochondrial 12S ribosomal RNA gene, and AUNA1 locus (13q14–21), were also found to be related to nonsyndromic AN (Table 1).

Some types of hereditary neurological disorders are known to be associated with AN, and these include Charcot–Marie–Tooth disease, Friedreich's ataxia, Refsum syndrome, Mohr–Tranebjaerg syndrome, mitochondrial disease, and autosomal dominant optic atrophy (ADOA). Recent progress in genetics has changed the classification of these neurological disorders. Details about subtypes of neurological disorders in association with AN are now becoming clear. As an instance, *peripheral myelin protein 22* (*PMP22*), *myelin protein zero* (*MPZ*), *gap junction protein beta-1* (*GJB1*), *early growth response 2* (*EGR2*), and *N-myc downstream regulated gene* (*NDRG1*) were found as the genes causing Charcot–Marie–Tooth disease [6]. *PMP22*, *MPZ*, and *NDRG1*, at least, have been reported to be associated with AN.

Epidemiology of Genetic AN

The prevalence of AN in children with severe or profound hearing loss has been reported to be 7% to 15%. AN occurs in bilateral ears in most patients. According to a study about the causes of AN, 42% of patients are associated with hereditary neurological disorders, 10% with toxic, metabolic, immunological, and infectious causes (anoxia, hyperbilirubinemia, drug reaction, demyelination, viral infection), and 48% with no known causes [3]. Many nonsyndromic AN cases with no known causes probably have a genetic basis. The inheritance pattern of such AN is mostly sporadic or autosomal recessive [4], rarely X-linked or autosomal dominant.

Pathophysiology, Diagnosis, and Treatment for Genetic AN

Pathophysiology

Because AN is diagnosed on the basis of audiological test results showing normal function of outer hair cells and impairment of auditory neurons, the pathophysiology of AN may be impairment of synapses in inner hair cells, auditory neurons, or both. In addition, impairment of central auditory pathways may be associated with such disorders. Hearing loss caused by impairment of inner hair cells is not compatible with the term "auditory neuropathy." However, impairment of inner hair cells is usually referred to as auditory neuropathy because current clinical tests cannot discriminate impairment of synapses in inner hair cells and auditory neurons.

Among nonsyndromic AN, some mutations in the *OTOF* gene cause impairment of inner hair cells [7], some mutations in the pejvakin gene may cause impairment of the organ of Corti and peripheral and central auditory neurons [5], and some mutations in the *GJB2* gene may cause impairment of inner hair cells and nerve endings beneath the hair cells. Among syndromic AN, studies on temporal bones from Friedreich's ataxia and Charcot–Marie–Tooth disease showed degeneration of spiral ganglion cells with or without degeneration of inner hair cells and demyelination of auditory neurons. A recent study on the temporal bones from an AN patient having a mutation in the *MPZ* gene revealed prominent loss of spiral ganglion cells and auditory neurons, and incomplete remyelination, as well as almost normal inner and outer hair cells. In this patient, detailed audiological evaluation demonstrated that hearing loss is mainly caused by decreased auditory input through a diminished number of auditory neurons [8].

Diagnosis

In clinical diagnosis of genetic AN, patients first undergo audiological evaluation to detect AN, followed by otological, genetic, and neurological evaluation of the etiology of AN. For audiological evaluation, diagnosis of sensorineural hearing loss is made by pure tone audiometry. A loss of speech comprehension that is out of proportion with pure tone hearing thresholds raises a suspicion of AN. Identification of preserved outer hair cell function by transient evoked otoacoustic emissions (TEOAE) or distortion product otoacoustic emissions (DPOAE), and confirmation of absent or prominently abnormal auditory brainstem response (ABR), lead to the diagnosis of AN. For diagnosis of etiology, patients or parents of AN children are first carefully asked about nongenetic factors, that is, risk factors during pregnancy, delivery, and neonatal and infantile periods such as anoxia, hyperbilirubinemia, prematurity, low birth weight, use of drugs, demyelinating disorders, or viral infection. Then, hereditary neurological disorders such as Charcot–Marie–Tooth disease,

Friedreich's ataxia, and mitochondrial disease are evaluated by neurological examination to make diagnosis of syndromic AN or nonsyndromic AN. Genetic tests for appropriate genes are conducted to identify genetic cause after obtaining informed consent.

Treatment

There has been no fundamental treatment for AN. Thus, auditory rehabilitaton using hearing aids or cochlear implants plays a central role for most AN patients. However, hearing aids are not as effective in AN patients compared to non-AN patients with equivalent level of pure tone thresholds because of poor speech comprehension, which is a characteristic feature of AN. Furthermore, in general, cochlear implants have also been thought to be ineffective for AN patients because auditory neurons cannot respond correctly upon stimulation. However, this is not the case for AN caused by *OTOF* gene mutations because the auditory neurons are normal in this type of AN. Theoretically, a cochlear implant, which directly stimulates auditory neurons within the cochlea, should be effective in AN caused by *OTOF* gene mutations. In fact, successful results of cochlear implants have been reported in this type of AN [4,9]. Cochlear implant was also reported to be effective for a family with AN mapping to the AUNA1 locus.

Representative Genes Causing Nonsyndromic Auditory Neuropathy

OTOF Gene

The *OTOF* gene is the first gene identified as the cause of nonsyndromic AN. The *OTOF* gene was originally found as a locus (DFNB9: 2p22–23) that is linked to autosomal recessive, congenital, severe to profound hearing loss. Then, it was identified as a gene coding the cell membrane protein otoferlin, which is expressed in the cochlea, vestibule, and brain [10]. *OTOF* consists of 48 exons, and has multiple isoforms, by alternative splicing combined with the use of several translation initiation sites. Otoferlin belongs to a family of membrane-anchored cytosolic proteins containing six repeats of a structural module that binds calcium (the C2 domain), and they are involved in vesicle membrane fusion.

Mutant mice lacking otoferlin are profoundly deaf, with no detectable ABR across all sound frequencies tested. However, DPOAE show that outer hair cell function is maintained, as was seen in human AN patients. In these mice, the structure of the inner ear including hair cells and spiral ganglion cells is normal, but complete abolition of inner hair cell synaptic exocytosis in response to cell depolarization is detected, which is consistent with a failure of inner hair cell neurotransmitter release.

Genetic tests of *OTOF* gene were conducted in 65 American families with autosomal recessive nonsyndromic hearing loss, including 9 families with AN. Eight mutations that were related to hearing loss were found in 6 families, including 5 families with AN. One of these families, which had the I515T mutation, showed temperature-sensitive AN in which hearing loss is aggravated with elevation of body temperature and returns to mild hearing loss with normalization of the temperature. A nonsense mutation Q829X in *OTOF* gene was first identified in a Spanish population and was found in approximately 3% of autosomal recessive hearing loss in Spanish children, making it the third most frequent mutation in this population [11]. Later studies in other populations showed that the Q829X mutation also caused dysfunction of outer hair cells. Thus, it is necessary to explore the significance of this frequent mutation in both AN and non-AN sensorineural hearing loss.

Pejvakin gene

Pejvakin gene is the second gene to be identified as the cause of nonsyndromic AN [5]. This gene was identified in the DFNB59 (2q31.1-q31.3) locus by linkage analysis in two Iranian families with autosomal recessive, severe to profound, congenital hearing loss, in which T54I and R183W missense mutations were detected. Pejvakin protein consists of 352 amino acids, but its function has been unknown. Pejvakin protein is localized in the cochlear hair cells, supporting cells, spiral ganglion cells, and the first three relays of the central auditory pathway. On the other hand, dysfunction of outer hair cells was reported in a Moroccan family with insertion of T at 113–114 as well as in a Turkish family with homozygous nonsense mutation R167X and another Turkish family with homozygous missense mutation R183W which is the same mutation as in the Iranian family with non-syndromic AN. Furthermore, mutant mice that have an abnormal *pejvakin* gene demonstrated progressive hearing loss with or without the loss of otoacoustic emissions (OAE), depending on the mutation introduced in the pejvakin gene. These findings indicate that the *pejvakin* gene may cause both AN and non-AN sensorineural hearing loss, depending on the type of mutation and different background factors.

Representative Genes Causing Syndromic Auditory Neuropathy

Charcot–Marie–Tooth Disease

Charcot–Marie–Tooth disease is the most common hereditary peripheral neuropathy, characterized by slowly progressive weakness, muscle atrophy, and sensory impairment, all most marked in the distal part of the legs. Charcot–Marie–Tooth disease is classified into subtypes based on clinical features and causative genes, and hearing loss has been known to be associated with some of these subtypes. Recently, AN was found in some of such Charcot–Marie–Tooth disease patients with hearing loss and established as a syndromic AN. The following three subtypes of Charcot–Marie–Tooth disease have been reported in association with syndromic AN.

Mutations in *PMP22* genes cause the CMT1A subtype of Charcot–Marie–Tooth disease, which shows autosomal dominant inheritance. PMP22 protein encoded by *PMP22* gene is a cell membrane protein that consists of approximately 5% of components of myelin sheath. AN has been reported in an American CMT1A family in which the A67P mutation was identified [12].

Mutations in the *MPZ* gene cause the CMT1B subtype of Charcot–Marie–Tooth disease, which shows autosomal dominant inheritance. MPZ protein coded by *MPZ* gene is a glycoprotein specific to Schwann cells, consists of approximately 50% myelin sheath components, and constitutes the myelin sheath as a complex with myelin basic protein and PMP22 protein. AN with an onset after 40 years of age has been reported in an American CMT1B family in which the Y145S mutation was identified. A study of temporal bone pathology in one member of this family revealed prominent loss of spiral ganglion cells and auditory neurons as well as well-preserved inner and outer hair cells [8].

Mutation in the *NDRG1* gene causes the CMT4D subtype of Charcot–Marie–Tooth disease, which shows autosomal recessive inheritance [13]. The *NDRG1* gene is highly expressed in Schwann cells and is expected to play a role in inhibition of mitosis and promotion of differentiation. R148X mutation in the *NDRG1* gene was identified in many European families in which AN was also found. In a CMT4D family, 25 of 39 family members complained of hearing loss that developed between 13 and 26 years of age.

Autosomal Dominant Optic Atrophy (ADOA) with Sensorineural Deafness

ADOA is a dominantly inherited disorder characterized by symmetrical optic atrophy, central visual impairment, and color vision defect. Although ADOA generally appears as an isolated disorder, it is sometimes associated with sensorineural deafness. Furthermore, some ADOA patients may be associated with not only sensorineural deafness but also several other phenotypes such as ataxia and peripheral neuropathy. Mutations in the *OPA1* gene have been found in a majority of patients with ADOA, and such mutations have also been reported in ADOA with sensorineural deafness and ADOA with deafness and other phenotypes.

The *OPA1* gene encodes a dynamin-related GTPase, which is targeted to mitochondria by an N-terminus import sequence motif and is anchored to the inner ear membrane facing the intermembrane space [14,15]. OPA1 protein is involved in the regulation of mitochondrial fusion and remodeling of mitochondrial cristae, the apoptotic process through the control of cytochrome C redistribution, and the maintenance of mitochondrial DNA [16]. The OPA1 protein is expressed in all tissues examined, but most strongly in the retina and brain. In the ear, OPA1 protein was found to be widely expressed in the sensory and neural cochlear cells. Although the exact pathological mechanism is unknown, an abnormality of the OPA1 protein may cause an abnormality of the mitochondria, leading to insufficient energy support. This lack could then result in a dysfunction of axoplasmic transport in the nerve fibers.

In patients with ADOA and sensorineural deafness, AN was first identified in two subjects by audiological evaluation including OAE and ABR in a study of five subjects from four families having this disorder [17]. Skin fibroblasts from these subjects showed hyperfragmentation of the mitochondrial network, decreased mitochondrial membrane potential, and ATP synthesis defect, indicating that AN in these patients may be related to energy defects caused by a fragmented mitochondrial network.

References

1. Kaga K, Nakamura M, Shinogami M, et al (1996) Auditory nerve disease of both ears revealed by auditory brainstem responses, electrocochleography and otoacoustic emissions. Scand Audiol 25:233–238
2. Starr A, Picton TW, Sininger Y, et al (1996) Auditory neuropathy. Brain 119:741–753
3. Starr A, Sininger YS, Pratt H, et al (2000) The varieties of auditory neuropathy. J Basic Clin Physiol Pharmacol 11:215–230
4. Varga R, Kelley PM, Keats BJ, et al (2003) Non-syndromic recessive auditory neuropathy is the result of mutations in the otoferlin (OTOF) gene. J Med Genet 40:45–50
5. Delmaghani S, del Castillo FJ, Michel V, et al (2006) Mutations in the gene encoding pejvakin, a newly identified protein of the afferent auditory pathway, cause DFNB59 auditory neuropathy. Nat Genet 38:770–778
6. Boerkoel CF, Takashima H, Garcia CA, et al (2002) Charcot-Marie-Tooth disease and related neuropathies: mutation distribution and genotype-phenotype correlation. Ann Neurol 51: 190–201
7. Roux I, Safieddine S, Nouvian R, et al (2006) Otoferlin, defective in a human deafness form, is essential for exocytosis at the auditory ribbon synapse. Cell 127:277–289
8. Starr A, Michalewski HJ, Zeng F, et al (2003) Pathology and physiology of auditory neuropathy with a novel mutation in the MPZ gene (Tyr145->Ser). Brain 126:1604–1619
9. Rouillon I, Marcolla A, Roux I, et al (2006) Results of cochlear implantation in two children with mutations in the OTOF gene. Int J Pediatr Otorhinolaryngol 70:689–696
10. Yasunaga S, Grati M, Cohen-Salmon M, et al (1999) A mutation in OTOF, encoding otoferlin, a FER-1-like protein, causes DFNB9, a nonsyndromic form of deafness. Nat Genet 21:363–369
11. Migliosi V, Modamio-Hoybjor S, Moreno-Pelayo MA, et al (2002) Q829X, a novel mutation in the gene encoding otoferlin (OTOF), is frequently found in Spanish patients with prelingual non-syndromic hearing loss. J Med Genet 39:502–506
12. Kovach MJ, Lin J, Boyadjiev S, et al (1999) A unique point mutation in the PMP22 gene is associated with Charcot-Marie-Tooth disease and deafness. Am J Hum Genet 64: 1580–1593
13. Kalaydjieva L, Gresham D, Gooding R, et al (2000) N-myc downstream-regulated gene 1 is mutated in hereditary motor and sensory neuropathy-Lom. Am J Hum Genet 67:47–58

14. Delettre C, Lenaers G, Griffoin J, et al (2000) Nuclear gene OPA1, encoding a mitochondrial dynamin-related protein, is mutated in dominant optic atrophy. Nat Genet 26:207–210
15. Alexander C, Votruba M, Pesch UEA, et al (2000) OPA1, encoding a dynamin-related GTPase, is mutated in autosomal dominant optic atrophy linked to chromosome 3q28. Nat Genet 26:211–215
16. Zeviani M (2008) OPA1 mutations and mitochondrial DNA damage: keeping the magic in shape. Brain 131:314–317
17. Amati-Bonneau P, Guichet A, Olichon A, et al (2005) OPA1 R445H mutation in optic atrophy associated with sensorineural deafness. Ann Neurol 58:958–963

Part III
Cochlear Implants

Environmental Sound Perception in Patients with Cochlear Implants Compared with That in Patients with Auditory Nerve Diseases (Auditory Neuropathy) and Cortical Deafness

Kimitaka Kaga[1] and Yusuke Akamatsu[2]

Summary

The mechanism for perception of environmental sounds is considered to be different from the cognitive mechanism of language. The environmental sound perception of cochlear implantees appears to be good but not perfect. However, its underlying mechanism is not yet known. The aim of this study was to investigate perception of environmental sounds in postlingually deaf patients with cochlear implants compared with that in patients with central auditory disorders. Seventeen postlingual patients with cochlear implants, 6 patients with auditory nerve disease (auditory neuropathy), and 10 patients with cortical deafness were selected for the comparison. A tape-recorded environmental sound perception test of 24 environmental sounds, which was developed by the authors in 1987, was used. This test is divided into two categories: the category of vocalization includes human voice as well as animal and bird sounds, and the category of non-voice sounds includes sounds of nature and musical instruments, as well as sounds from man-made sources. The test procedure consists of two steps. The first step (open set) is only to listen and to identify each sound either orally or in writing. The second step (closed set) is to listen and chooses a picture card matching test form among four different pictures. The percentages of correctly identified environmental sounds in postlingually deaf patients with cochlear implants was markedly higher than that in patients with cortical deafness, but was similar to that in patients with auditory nerve disease (auditory neuropathy), in both the closed and open sets. Our study revealed that the perception of environmental sounds in postlingual patients with cochlear implants was not good in the open set but markedly better in the closed set. This result is similar to those for auditory nerve disease patients but completely different from those for cortical deafness patients. The ability of patients with cochlear implants to perceive environmental sounds is similar to that of patients

[1]National Institute of Sensory Organs, National Tokyo Medical Center, 2-5-1 Higashigaoka, Meguro-ku, Tokyo 152-8902, Japan
[2]Department of Otolaryngology, and Head and Neck Surgery, The University of Tokyo, Tokyo, Japan

doi: 10.1007/978-4-431-09433-3_6, © Springer 2009

with auditory nerve disease, perhaps because information carried by the cochlear nerve is similarly degraded.

Key words Environmental sounds, Postlingual deafness, Cochlear implant, Auditory neuropathy, Cortical deafness

Introduction

Occasionally, during a routine clinical evaluation of auditory-evoked brainstem responses (ABR), abnormalities are encountered in which there is no ABR to intense click stimulation but the patients show normal or a mild hearing loss with preservation of otoacoustic emissions (OAEs) and summating potentials in electrocochleography. Most of these patients complain of mild hearing impairment and difficulty in understanding speech, partially when using the telephone. Using two particular tests of auditory function, ABRs and OAEs, we are able to determine that the auditory nerve function is abnormal, whereas the cochlear function (at least as far as the outer hair cells) is intact. These features are consistent with a peculiar system of auditory dysfunction described as auditory nerve disease or auditory neuropathy in 1996 [1,2]. According to a widely accepted view, in most cases this disorder results from an impaired function of the auditory nerve caused by demyelination and, to a lesser extent, by axonal loss [1–5]. Cochlear implantation in children diagnosed with auditory neuropathy is reported to be highly effective in most cases because each child showed improved listening and communication skills that enabled each child to take advantage of different communication and educational options. Implantation has been less successful in a child with postlingual onset of Friedreich's ataxia, in which there is loss of neurons [6]. No other cases of cochlear implantation in patients with postlingual auditory nerve disease have been reported.

In nearly all postlingually deafened individuals who receive cochlear implants, the primary deficit is loss of hair cells, although there may well be loss of neurons as well. In spite of the different site of lesion, these individuals share with those having auditory neuropathy the task of deciphering signals form the auditory nerve that are far from normal.

The mechanism for perception of environmental sounds is considered to be different from the cognitive mechanism of language in the brain. The perception of environmental sounds in cochlear implantees with postlingual deafness appears to be fair or good. However, perception of environmental sounds with cochlear implants has been little studied compared with speech sound perception. On the other hand, in central auditory disorders, the perception of environmental sounds is damaged differently, caused by influenced levels of the central auditory pathway.

The aim of this study is to investigate the perception of environmental sounds in cochlear implantees compared with that in patients with auditory neuropathy (auditory nerve disease) and cortical deafness.

Table 1. Profile of patients

Patients	Number	Age (years)	Affected site	Etiology
a Cochlear implant	17	14–75 (X = 50.24; SD = 18.35)	Inner and outer hair cells	Sensory hearing loss
b Auditory neuropathy (auditory nerve disease)	6	5–68 (X = 40.67; SD = 22.38)	Auditory nerve	Unknown
c Cortical deafness (auditory agnosia)	10	22–75 (X = 51.80; SD = 22.28)	Auditory cortex or auditory radiation	Cerebrovascular accidents

Subjects and Methods

Subjects were 17 postlingually deaf patients with cochlear implants. Also studied were 6 patients with auditory neuropathy, with normal distortion product otoacoustic emission (DPOAE) but absent auditory brainstem responses and compound action potentials of electrocochleography (ECochG); and 10 patients with cortical deafness (auditory agnosia), whose bilateral auditory cortices or auditory radiation were lesioned because of cerebrovascular accidents. Profiles of the three groups are presented in Table 1.

An environmental sound perception test of 24 environmental sounds, which was developed by Kaga and Sugishita in 1987 [7], was used (Table 2). This test is divided into two categories: the category of vocalizations includes human voice, and animal and bird sounds, and the category of non-voice sound includes sounds of nature and of musical instruments, and sounds from manmade sources. The test procedure consists of two steps. The first step (open set) is only to listen and identify the correct sound by giving either an oral or a written answer. The second step (closed set) is a picture-matching test in which patients are requested to choose the correct answer card among four different picture cards. In normal subjects, the percentage of correct answers in the open and closed set is 100%. In Fig. 1, sound spectrograms of 24 test sounds are shown.

Results

As shown in Fig. 2, the cochlear implant patients correctly identified only half the sounds in the open-set task, a performance similar to that the auditory neuropathy subjects (no significant differences between groups). The cortically deaf individuals performed far worse than either of the other group ($P < 001$). All groups performed better on the close-set picture-pointing task, but again there was no significant

Table 2. Data sheet of environmental sound perception test

Test of environmental sound perception	**Naming**	**Picture matching**
Trumpet		
Telephone ring		
Mewing (cat)		
Cawing (crow)		
Drum		
Man's voice		
Whistle of wind		
Mooing (cow)		
Electric train		
Barking (dog)		
Woman's voice		
Car		
Wall clock		
Wave		
Singing		
Neighing (horse)		
Baby's cry		
English speech		
Murmuring of a stream		
Gunshot		
Crowing (cock)		
Saw		
Laughter		
Footsteps		

Date

No.

Name **Age** ( )

Diagnosis

Onset

Results

Naming: %

Picture matching: %

difference between the cochlear implant and auditory neuropathy groups, and each of theses groups was far superior to the cortical deafness group ($P < 001$).

Further comparisons were made between the auditory neuropathy and cochlear implant groups because their overall performance was so similar (Fig. 3). In the open-set task, the scores were somewhat better for the vocalization than the non-vocalization sounds. Of note, the two groups are similar on each of these subtests. All differences were small for the closed-set task where all scores were near 100%.

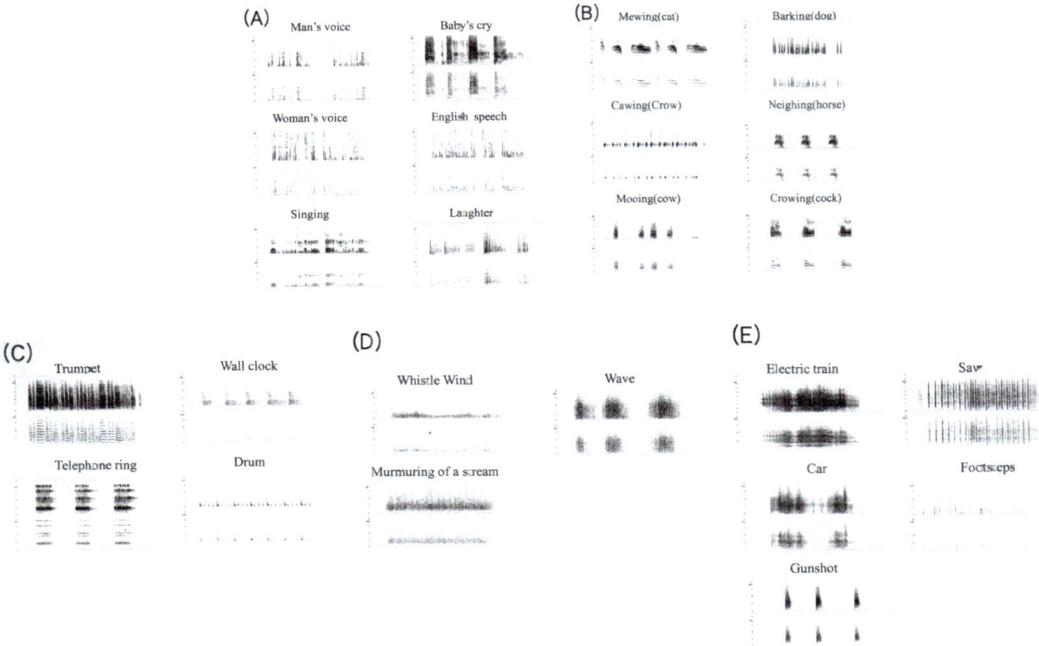

Fig. 1. Analysis of sound spectrograms of 24 items in environmental sound perception test: **A, B** categories of vocalizations; **C–E** categories of nonvocal sounds (non-voice)

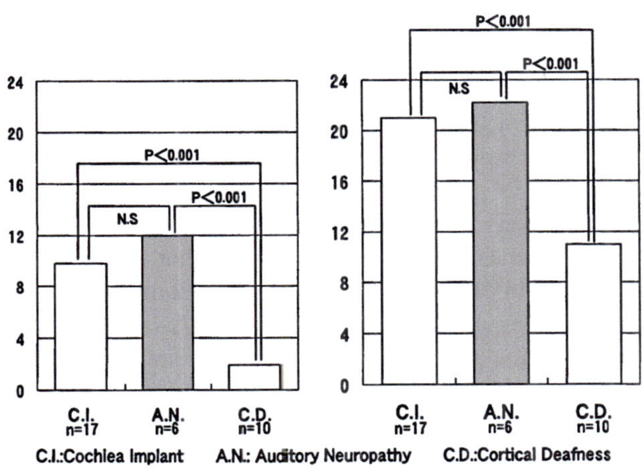

Fig. 2. Mean and standard deviation of total correct answers in open (*left*) and closed (*right*) sets of three groups in the bar graph: patients with cochlear implants (*C.I.*), auditory nerve disease (*A.N.*), and cortical deafness (*C.D.*)

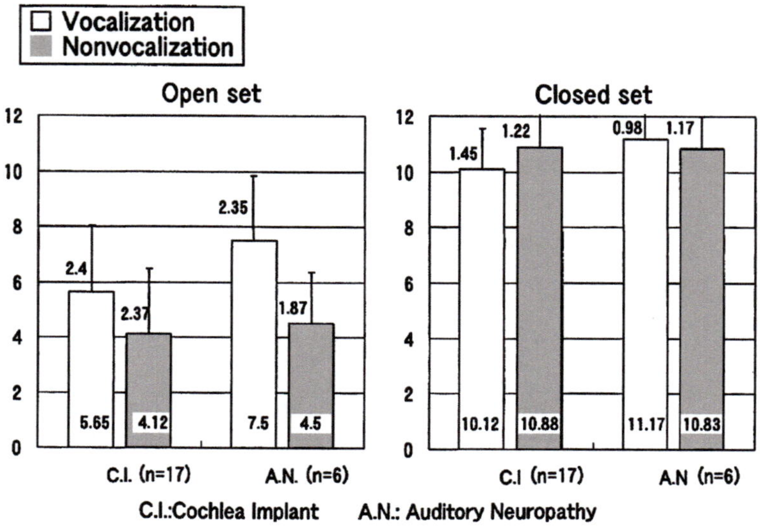

Fig. 3. Mean and standard deviation of total answers in open set (*left*) and closed set (*right*) of voice (*open bars*) and non-voice (*shaded bars*) categories in patients with cochlear implants and auditory neuropathy

Discussion

Our study revealed that the perception of environmental sounds by postlingually deaf patients with cochlear implants is not perfect even in the closed set, and it is quite similar to the performance of individuals with auditory neuropathy. However, it is clear that patients with cochlear implants are completely different from patients with cortical deafness, with far better perception. This result demonstrates that the auditory mechanism in patients with a cochlear implant has a certain limitation regarding perception of environmental sounds. The perceptive ability of environmental sounds in patients with cochlear implants is similar to auditory neuropathy but completely different from cortical deafness. This finding suggests that the perceptive mechanism of the cochlear implant is not cognitive disorder, but a deficiency in the information conveyed by the auditory nerve.

The common features of these sounds were impulsive and repetitive. In the open-set task, most of the patients could not identify sounds of a horse, a stream, or a car, which may be due to a lack of distinctive feature of these noises. Performance was much improved in the closed-set condition, where the available cues perhaps allowed the wrong choices to be excluded as much as they allowed the correct choice to be recognized.

The similarity between the auditory neuropathy and cochlear implant groups is remarkable. In the case of auditory neuropathy, the impaired identification of environmental sounds, similar to the impaired perception of speech, may be attributed to the impoverished representation of hair cell activity by the auditory nerve; timing information is lost, and intensity information is probably poorly represented. In the cochlear implant patients, neuron loss may play a role, but also the cochlear implant itself is limited in the amount of information that is conveyed to the auditory nerve.

Acknowledgments This work was supported by a Grant for Research on Sensory and Communicative Disorders (H18-Kankakuki-general-003) from the Ministry of Health, Labour and Welfare, and by a Grant-in-Aid for Scientific Research from Areas (A)(2)-15209055 from the Ministry of Education, Culture, Sports Science and Technology of Japan.

References

1. Kaga K, Nakamura M, Shinogami M, et al (1996) Auditory nerve disease of both ears revealed by auditory brainstem responses, electrocochleography and otoacoustic emissions. Scand Audiol 25:233–238
2. Star A, Picton PW, Sininger Y, et al (1996) Auditory neuropathy. Brain 119:741–753
3. Starr A, Sininger Y, Nguyen T, et al (2006) Cochlear receptor (microphonic and summating potentials, otoacoustic emissions) and auditory pathway (auditory brain stem potentials) activity in auditory neuropathy. Ear Hear 22:91–99
4. Butinar D, Zidar J, Leonardis L, et al (1999) Hereditary auditory, vestibular, motor and sensory neuropathy in a Slovenian Roma (Gypsy) kindred. Ann Neurol 46:36–44
5. Sheykholeslami K, Kaga K, Kaga M (2001) An isolated and sporadic auditory neuropathy (auditory nerve disease): report of five patients. J Laryngol Otol 115:530–534
6. Miyamoto RT, Kirk KI, Renshaw J, et al (1999) Cochlear implantation in auditory neuropathy. Laryngoscope 109:181–185
7. Kaga K, Shindo M, Tanaka Y (1997) Central auditory information processing in patients with bilateral auditory cortex lesions. Acta Otolaryngol Suppl 532:77–82

Pediatric Cochlear Implantation in Auditory Neuropathy

Lee-Suk Kim and Sung-Wook Jeong

Summary

Auditory neuropathy (AN) is a hearing disorder caused by desynchronized neural discharges of the auditory nerve. Some reports have shown that cochlear implantation has been successful for rehabilitation of children with AN, and that their altered neural synchrony can be restored by electrical stimulation introduced by cochlear implants. Most recipients achieved open-set speech perception abilities and showed progressive improvements in their communication skills. One case-control study showed that there were no significant differences in speech perception abilities between a group with AN and a group without AN after cochlear implantation. Consistent with previous reports, nine children with AN who received cochlear implants at Dong-A University Hospital benefited considerably from cochlear implantation. Although most recipients have demonstrated positive outcomes, some children in published reports have shown very poor performance of minimal improvements in close-set speech perception and no improvements in open-set speech perception. Cochlear implantation is considered a useful tool for the rehabilitation of children with AN, but the procedure needs to be done after the parents are informed fully about the uncertainty of results until the prognosis for this procedure can be established firmly. Additional long-term follow-up studies including a large number of recipients and more basic research to reveal the underlying pathophysiology of AN is necessary to establish cochlear implantation as a standard treatment option for this disorder.

Key words Auditory neuropathy, Cochlear implantation, Children, Speech perception

Department of Otolaryngology—Head and Neck Surgery, College of Medicine, Dong-A University, 3-1 Dongdaeshin-dong, Seo-gu, Busan 602-715, Korea

doi: 10.1007/978-4-431-09433-3_7,

Introduction

The main discomfort of patients suffering auditory neuropathy (AN) is seriously compromised speech comprehension ability, which is associated with poor temporal resolution caused by desynchronized neural discharges of auditory nerve fibers [1–3]. Conventional hearing aids are of little benefit as neural synchrony is not restored by such amplification [2,4]. Cochlear implantation has been reported to be successful for rehabilitation of patients with AN [5–12]. Most patients showed significant improvements in speech perception abilities after implantation, and measures of the electrical compound action potential (ECAP) and electrical auditory brainstem response (EABR) demonstrated that synchronous neural discharges can be restored in response to electrical stimulation introduced by the cochlear implants. The purpose of this chapter is to describe the rationale to perform cochlear implantation in children with AN, and to review the published outcomes of the procedure and the experience of Dong-A University Hospital.

Rationale to Perform Cochlear Implantation in Patients with Auditory Neuropathy

Some authors have reported positive outcomes after cochlear implantation in children with AN. In particular, Peterson et al. demonstrated that there were no major differences in speech perception measures between patients with AN and patients with nonneuropathic sensorineural hearing loss (SNHL) after cochlear implantation [10]. Given that the diseased auditory nerve has been considered unsuitable for cochlear implantation because the site of electrical stimulation via a cochlear implant is the spiral ganglion cells, the question of how patients with AN who have pathology of the auditory nerve could benefit from cochlear implantation must be raised. For patients with lesions in the inner hair cells or at the synaptic junctions between the inner hair cells and dendrites, cochlear implantation can work because the signal introduced by the implant bypasses the site of the lesion. In fact, some reports showed that children with AN caused by a mutation in the OTOF gene, which leads to inner hair cell dysfunction, received considerable benefit from cochlear implantation [11,12]. However, if the lesions are in the auditory nerve itself, the auditory signal might not be propagated through the auditory nerve. About this point of view, some reports which have shown that patients with SNHL who are optimal candidates for cochlear implantation have true neuropathy of the auditory nerve and that electrical stimulation of a severely diseased auditory nerve can elicit synchronized neural activity need to be considered. Nadol et al. showed that the residual spiral ganglion cell population of patients with congenital or genetic sensorineural hearing loss was less than half of that in subjects with normal hearing [13]. Fayad et al. found that two implanted patients who showed average performances had only 10% of the normal number of spiral ganglion cells [14].

Shepherd et al. showed that clear EABR waveforms could be obtained from a cat with extensive neural pathology (less than 5% of spiral ganglion survival) [15], and Zhou et al. showed that electrical stimulation of the auditory nerve in myelin-deficient mice could evoke EABR [16]. There are a few similar findings of spiral ganglion cell loss with auditory nerve degeneration and preserved organ of Corti in postmortem temporal bone histological studies of patients with AN [17,18]. Moreover, patients with deafness induced by hereditary sensory motor neuropathy type 1A, which causes peripheral demyelinating neuropathy, have been reported to show significant improvements in speech discrimination after cochlear implantation [19].

Cochlear implantation is a rational option for patients among whom limited or no benefit is obtained from appropriate auditory rehabilitation using an optimally fitted low-gain hearing aid. However, the pathophysiology of AN needs to be understood more clearly if we are to offer cochlear implantations to patients with AN with more confidence.

Reported Outcomes of Cochlear Implantation in Children with Auditory Neuropathy

There are several reports on the results of cochlear implantation in children with AN [5–12,20–22] (Tables 1, 2). Most children achieved open-set speech perception abilities and showed progressive improvements in communication skills. Some children achieved the ability to have telephone conversations. One case-control study showed that there were no significant differences in postoperative speech perception abilities between a group with AN and a group without AN [10]. By contrast, two reports showed limited benefits after cochlear implantation [20,21]. It is difficult to establish the factors contributing to postoperative performance from the literature. However, if it is supposed that unique features among poor performers that are not common in good performers are contributing factors of poor performance, some factors, including severe preoperative hearing loss and other neuropathies causing ataxia or blindness, might be involved. Two reports showed that outcomes following cochlear implantation in children with AN could be predicted by electrophysiology and imaging study. Gibson et al. reported that 75% of children with AN had a normal EABR and that their postoperative outcome was statistically better than a control group of deaf children; on the other hand, 25% of children with AN had an abnormal EABR and only gained limited benefit from a cochlear implant [22]. Walton et al. reported that 28% of children with AN had a cochlear nerve deficiency revealed by magnetic resonance imaging (MRI) and that children with AN with a cochlear nerve deficiency also tended to have an abnormal EABR and poor postoperative outcomes [23].

Cochlear implantation is a viable option for children with AN who receive limited or no benefit from conservative management, and good results can be

Table 1. Preoperative characteristics of implanted children with auditory neuropathy in published reports

First author	Pt no.	Onset of HL	PTA (dB)	Risk factors of AN	Additional diagnosis
Rance 1999 [20]	1	Birth	115	prema./bili.	
Miyamoto 1999 [21]	1	Birth, progressive[a]	97		Friedreich's ataxia, blindness
Trautwein 2000 [5]	1	Birth	100		
Shallop 2001 [6]	5	Birth	Severe to profound		
Buss 2002 [7]	4	Birth	94–103		Mondini deformity (1)[b]
Madden 2002 [8]	4	Birth			
Mason 2003 [9]	2	Birth		prema./bili. (1)[a]	
Peterson 2003 [10]	10	Birth	50–105 (9)[b], 130 (1)[b]		
Rouillon 2006 [12]	2	Birth			OTOF mutation
Gibson 2007 [22]	60				

Pt, patient; HL, hearing loss; PTA, pure tone average; AN, auditory neuropathy; prema., prematurity; bili., hyperbilirubinemia
[a] Deaf at age of 10.6 years
[b] Number within parentheses indicates the numbers of patients

expected from cochlear implantation in most recipients. However, some children with possible signs of true neuropathy of the cochlear nerve, such as peripheral neuropathy, abnormal EABR findings, and cochlear nerve deficiency on MRI, could have poor postoperative outcomes. Further investigations to reveal the prognostic factors and more long-term follow-up studies of a large number of subjects should be gathered to establish whether cochlear implantation can be offered as a standard treatment method for children with AN.

Cochlear Implantation in Children with Auditory Neuropathy: Experience of Dong-A University Hospital

Nine children with AN received cochlear implantation at a mean age of 4 years (range, 1 year 9 months to 11 years 5 months) at Dong-A University Hospital between May 2002 and November 2005. The mean age at diagnosis of AN was 1 year 7 months (range, 5 months to 5 years 4 months). Five of the children were boys and four were girls. Three of the children had cognitive disorders including mild mental retardation and mild pervasive developmental disorder.

All the children benefited considerably from cochlear implantation. Their aided pure tone thresholds were 40 dB or better. Good ECAP or EABR results were

Table 2. Postoperative characteristics and speech perception outcomes of implanted children with auditory neuropathy in the published literature

First author	Pt no.	Mean age (years) at surgery	Device	EABR	NRT	CI-PTA (dB)	Speech perception outcomes
Rance 1999 [20]	1	3.8	Nucleus	NR			CS, chance level; OS, 8% on PBK
Miyamoto 1999 [21]	1	10.9				39	CS, mild improvement; OS, no improvement
Trautwein 2000 [5]	1	3.3	Nucleus		Yes	40	Significant improvement
Shallop 2001 [6]	5	4.7		Yes	Yes	25–40	Significant improvement/some, telephone use
Buss 2002 [7]	4	3.9	Clarion			26–39	Within 1 SD of control group mean
Madden 2002 [8]	4	2.1					Significant improvement
Mason 2003 [9]	2	2.1		Yes		15, 35	IT MAIS, 34/40 (1)[a]
Peterson 2003 [10]	10	5.3	Nucleus (9)[a] Clarion (1)[a]	Yes	Yes	<40	No difference from control group in MAIS score
Rouillon 2006 [12]	2	3.5	Nucleus		Yes	37, 45	OS word, 50%–100%; OS sentence, 40%–60%
Gibson 2007 [22]	60		Nucleus	Normal (75%) Abnormal (25%)			Children with normal EABR had significantly better outcome than control group

EABR, electrical auditory brainstem response; NRT, neural response telemetry; CI-PTA, pure tone average wearing cochlear implant; NR, no response; CS, close-set speech perception test; OS, open-set speech perception test; PBK, phonetically balanced kindergarten test; SD, standard deviation; IT MAIS, Infant Toddler Meaningful Auditory Integration Scale

[a]Number within parentheses indicates numbers of patients

obtained in all children, indicating that neural synchrony was restored by the electrical stimulation provided by the cochlear implant (Fig. 1). All children except one with a pervasive developmental disorder achieved open-set speech perception abilities.

The postoperative speech performances of these 9 children with AN were compared with those of 18 children with nonneuropathic SNHL who also received cochlear implants. The two groups were matched for variables including onset of hearing loss, age at implantation, duration of implant use, primary mode of communication, and proportion of subjects with cognitive disorders (Table 3). Postoperative speech performance was measured by the Categories of Auditory Performance, Monosyllabic Word test for phonemes, and the Common Phrases test. Children in both groups showed significant improvements in their speech perception abilities after implantation ($P < 0.01$). Postoperative speech perception abilities of the AN group were not significantly different from those of the control group ($P = 0.403$–0.932). These results show that the speech perception abilities of these children with AN are comparable to those of the children with SNHL following cochlear implantation (Fig. 2).

Considerations Before Deciding Cochlear Implantation

Patients with AN can have any degree of hearing ranging from normal hearing to profound hearing loss, and their auditory capacity may not be consistent. Some

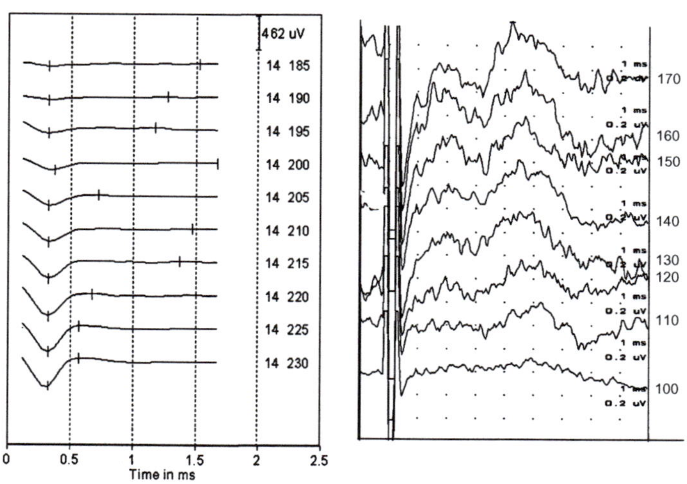

Fig. 1. Electrical compound action potential (*left*) and electrical auditory brainstem response (*right*) recorded from 21-month-old boy at electrodes no. 14 and 20, respectively. The current level for each trace is indicated on the *right*

Table 3. Matching data for comparison of speech performance outcomes

	Patients with auditory neuropathy ($n = 9$)	Patients with sensorineural hearing loss ($n = 18$)	P
Onset of hearing loss	All congenital	All congenital	
Age at implantation (years)	4.02 ± 3.18[a]	4.39 ± 2.88[a]	0.762*
Duration of implant use (years)	1.89 ± 0.74[a]	1.89 ± 0.74[a]	1.000*
Mode of communication (oral : nonverbal)	8 : 1	17 : 1	1.000**
Proportion of subjects with cognitive disorders	33% (3/9)	33% (6/18)	1.000**

[a] Values are presented as mean and standard deviation
* Independent t test; ** Fisher's exact test

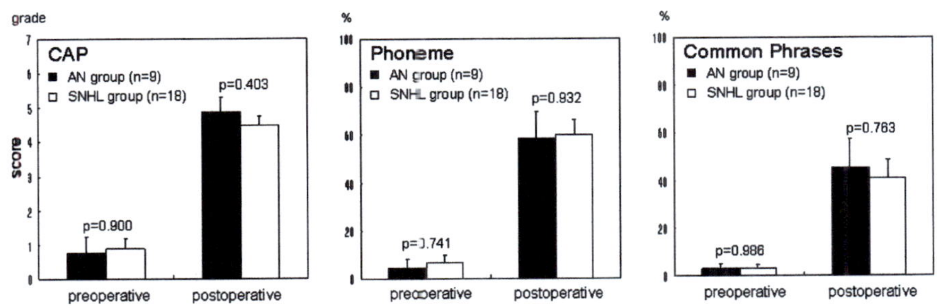

Fig. 2. Auditory performance of children with auditory neuropathy (AN) and those with non-neuropathic sensorineural hearing loss (SNHL). Scores are presented as mean and standard error. There were no statistically significant differences between the two groups in postoperative speech perception abilities,which were measured by using the Categories of Auditory Performance (*CAP*) (Mann–Whitney test, $P = 0.403$) and two open-set speech perception tests, namely, Monosyllabic Word test for *Phoneme* (independent t test, $P = 0.932$) and *Common Phrases* test (independent t test, $P = 0.763$)

young children with AN demonstrate spontaneous hearing improvement to a level with no need of amplification, show appearance of a normal auditory brainstem response (ABR), and develop speech and language normally without any intervention [4,8,24]. Spontaneous recovery has occurred in children under the age of 1 year and 6 months. Therefore, very young children or infants with AN should be assessed repeatedly for auditory capacity, speech development, and electrophysiological measures including ABR and otoacoustic emission to confirm the presence of persistent AN without spontaneous recovery before deciding to perform cochlear implantation. Although most reports are positive at present, implantation should be done only after the parents are informed fully about the uncertainty of results, because the prognosis for this procedure has not been firmly established.

Conclusions

Cochlear implantation is a useful tool for the rehabilitation of children with AN in cases in which no spontaneous improvements in hearing thresholds appear and where limited or no benefit is obtained from appropriate auditory rehabilitation using an optimally fitted low-gain hearing aid.

References

1. Starr A, McPherson D, Patterson J, et al (1991) Absence of both auditory evoked potentials and auditory percepts dependent on timing cues. Brain 114:1157–1180
2. Sininger Y, Hood LJ, Starr A, et al (1995) Hearing loss due to auditory neuropathy. Audiol Today 7:10–13
3. Starr A, Picton TW, Sininger Y, et al (1996) Auditory neuropathy. Brain 119:741–753
4. Berlin CI, Hood L, Morlet T, et al (2003) Auditory neuropathy/dys-synchrony: management and results in 193 patients. Presented at the 26th Annual Mid Winter Research Meeting of the Association for Research in Otolaryngology, Daytona Beach, FL, February 22–27, 2003
5. Trautwein PG, Sininger YS, Nelson R (2000) Cochlear implantation of auditory neuropathy. J Am Acad Audiol 11:309–315
6. Shallop JK, Peterson A, Facer GW, et al (2001) Cochlear implants in five cases of auditory neuropathy: postoperative findings and progress. Laryngoscope 111:555–562
7. Buss E, Labadie RF, Brown CJ, et al (2002) Outcome of cochlear implantation in pediatric auditory neuropathy. Otol Neurotol 23:328–332
8. Madden C, Rutter M, Hilbert L, et al (2002) Clinical and audiological features in auditory neuropathy. Arch Otolaryngol Head Neck Surg 128:1026–1030
9. Mason JC, De Michele A, Stevens C, et al (2003) Cochlear implantation in patients with auditory neuropathy of varied etiologies. Laryngoscope 113:45–49
10. Peterson A, Shallop J, Driscoll C, et al (2003) Outcomes of cochlear implantation in children with auditory neuropathy. J Am Acad Audiol 14:188–201
11. Loundon N, Marcolla A, Roux I, et al (2005) Auditory neuropathy or endocochlear hearing loss? Otol Neurotol 26:748–754
12. Rouillon I, Marcolla A, Roux I, et al (2006) Results of cochlear implantation in two children with mutations in the OTOF gene. Int J Pediatr Otorhinolaryngol 70:689–696
13. Nadol JB Jr, Young YS, Glynn RJ (1989) Survival of spiral ganglion cells in profound sensorineural hearing loss: implications for cochlear implantation. Ann Otol Rhinol Laryngol 98:411–416
14. Fayad J, Linthicum FH Jr, Otto SR, et al (1991) Cochlear implants: histopathologic findings related to performance in 16 human temporal bones. Ann Otol Rhinol Laryngol 100: 807–811
15. Shepherd RK, Javel E (1997) Electrical stimulation of the auditory nerve. I. Correlation of physiological responses with cochlear status. Hear Res 108:112–144
16. Zhou R, Abbas PJ, Assouline JG (1995) Electrically evoked auditory brainstem response in peripherally myelin-deficient mice. Hear Res 88:98–106
17. Spoendlin H (1974) Optic cochleovestibular degenerations in hereditary ataxias. II. Temporal bone pathology in two cases of Friedreich's ataxia with vestibulo-cochlear disorders. Brain 97:41–48
18. Starr A, Michalewski HJ, Zeng FG, et al (2003) Pathology and physiology of auditory neuropathy with a novel mutation in the MPZ gene (Tyr145->Ser). Brain 126:1604–1619

19. Postelmans JTF, Stokroos RJ (2006) Cochlear implantation in a patient with deafness induced by Charcot-Marie-Tooth disease (hereditary motor and sensory neuropathies). J Laryngol Otol 120:508–510
20. Rance G, Beer DE, Cone-Wesson B, et al (1999) Clinical findings for a group of infants and young children with auditory neuropathy. Ear Hear 20:238–252
21. Miyamoto RT, Kirk KI, Renshaw J, et al (1999) Cochlear implantation in auditory neuropathy. Laryngoscope 109:181–185
22. Gibson WP, Sanli H (2007) Auditory neuropathy: an update. Ear Hear 28:102S–106S
23. Walton J, Gibson WP, Sanli H, et al (2008) Predicting cochlear implant outcomes in children with auditory neuropathy. Otol Neurotol 29:302–309
24. Attias J, Raveh E (2007) Transient deafness in young candidates for cochlear implants. Audiol Neurootol 12:325–333

Cochlear Implantation for Children with Auditory Neuropathy Among Japanese Language Users

Kunihiro Fukushima[1], Yuko Kataoka[1], Yukihide Maeda[1], Shin Kariya[1], Susumu Tominaga[1], Rie Nagayasu[1], Akihiro Kawasaki[1], Shouichiro Fukuda[2], Naomi Toida[2], and Kazunori Nishizaki[1]

Summary

Among 80 prelingually deafened children who underwent cochlear implant at Okayama University Hospital, two auditory neuropathy/auditory dys-synchrony (AN/AD) cases with cochlear implant were identified from review of medical records. These two cases first demonstrated stable responses with distortion product otoacoustic emission, although later the response disappeared. In spite of the presence of AN/AD, the language development of these cases was quite satisfactory so far. Herein, we report the clinical course and language development of these auditory neuropathy cases with cochlear implant.

Key words Cochlear implant, Auditory neuropathy, Auditory dys-synchrony, Auditory nerve disease, Language development, OAE, Prelingual hearing loss

Introduction

Otoacoustic emission (OAE) is widely used in clinical practice [1]. Screenings based on the principles of OAE are being used during newborn hearing screening in various countries [2]. However, cases of children with actual hearing loss who exhibit normal responses on OAE screening have been reported [3–5], and these children may require more complicated postscreening diagnosis and face disruptions regarding the commencement of intervention, including the use of cochlear implants.

[1]Department of Otolaryngology Head and Neck Surgery, Okayama University Postgraduate School of Medicine, Dentistry and Pharmaceutical Science, 2-5-1 Shikata-cho, Okayama 700-8558, Japan

[2]Okayama Kanariya Gakuen, Okayama, Japan

doi: 10.1007/978-4-431-09433-3_8, © Springer 2009

Auditory neuropathy/neurodisease or auditory dys-synchrony (AN/AD) is a representative disorder in which favorable responses are obtained on OAE during screening [6,7]. Herein, we present the clinical courses of the children with OAE-positive hearing impairments and cochlear implants.

Patients and Methods

During 1990 to 2006, 80 children with prelingual hearing impairment underwent cochlear implantation at Okayama University Hospital, and positive responses on OAE were confirmed among 4 children. Although 2 of them had demonstrated transient reaction of positive distortion product otoacoustic emission (DPOAE) response at newborn hearing screening, we could not confirm the positive result at their first visit to our hospital.

The other two children were subjected to several audiological tests including unaided pure tone audiometry, sound field audiometry with cochlear implant, 57- or 67-type monosyllable speech perception tests [8], and developmental tests including WISC-III, WPPSI, or Kyoto developmental scale tests for Japanese language users [9]. Speech intelligibility was also evaluated by three audiologists separately when the children could speak voluntarily [10]. Picture vocabulary test (PVT) and reading comprehension test were also conducted [10].

Case Histories

Case 1

The patient was born after normal labor at 37 weeks of gestation in November 1999. Birth weight was 2750 g and Apgar score was 9/10. No family history of hearing impairment was documented, and there was no particular history during pregnancy. The patient was referred to our hospital for suspected hearing loss following the absence of responses on automated ABR at delivery. During ABR at the first visit, no responses were observed even at 100 dB nHL. However, DPOAE performed around the same time revealed responses within the normal range. The patient showed poor responses to sounds in the sound field. The use of hearing aids was initiated on both ears at 4 months postnatally. However, responses to sound were unfavorable even with hearing aids, and the aided threshold in the sound field was only 80 dB nHL. In addition, responses on DPOAE gradually decreased following the fitting of hearing aids.

Subsequent motor development was favorable. Cochlear implantation was performed on the left ear at 2 years postnatally in December 2001. Preoperative imaging, including computed tomography (CT) and magnetic resonance imaging (MRI), revealed no notable findings.

Following cochlear implantation, responses to sound rapidly improved (Fig. 1c), and language development also showed steady progress. Language development

Monosyllable speech perception test	
Consonant +vowel	88%
Vowel	100%
Speech intelligibility test	
	86%

WISC-III (CA 72M)	
VIQ	119
PIQ	129
Total IQ	126

Other language tests	
PVT (CA 6y0m)	6y9m
Reading comprehension test	4 (superior)
ITPA (CA 5y8m)	PLA 5-8

a) Language test results

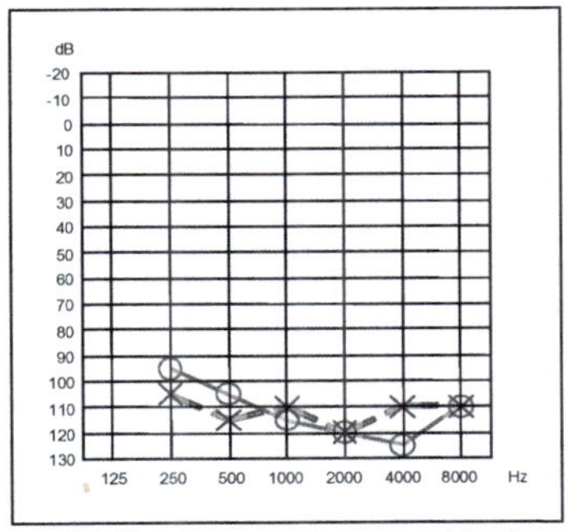

b) Postoperative, unaided

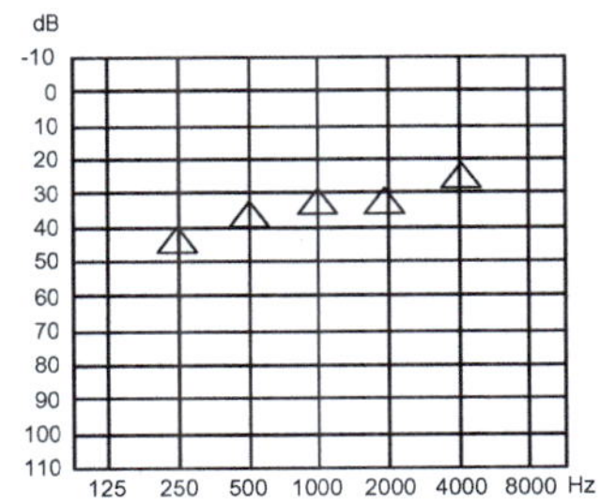

c) Postoperative, cochlear implant

Fig. 1. Case 1

of the case is summarized in Fig. 1a. The patient could use compound sentences and clauses in his daily diary when he was 6 years old. He is currently enrolled in a mainstream elementary school and participates in various school activities without problems.

Case 2

The patient was born by cesarean section at 38 weeks of gestation in May 2001. Birth weight was 2728 g and Apgar score was 9/10. Although no particular delays in motor development, such as head control, were observed thereafter, the patient received a consultation at another hospital because of a noticeable delay in language development at age 2. The patient was then referred to our hospital after ABR performed by the pediatric neurologist revealed hearing loss. A peepshow test indicated severe hearing impairment. Consequently, the patient received educational intervention at Kanariya School from the age of 2 years and 11 months, and immediately began wearing hearing aids on both ears. At this point, reexamination using DPOAE repeatedly confirmed positive responses. Although the use of hearing aids resulted in improved speech and gradual increases in vocabulary, a marked delay in language development was also observed. Therefore, at the age of 4 years, cochlear implantation was performed on the right ear in November 2005 (Fig. 2b). After 3 months use of cochlear implant, she complained of the invalidity of her

Monosyllable speech perception test	
Consonant +vowel	65%
Vowel	100%
Speech intelligibility test	
	50%

Kyoto developmental quotient	
Preoperative (CA 50M)	Cognitive 92 Language 74
Postoperative (CA 62M)	Cognitive 103 Language 92

WPPSI test (CA 67M)	
VIQ	70
PIQI	98
Total IQ	80

a) Language test results

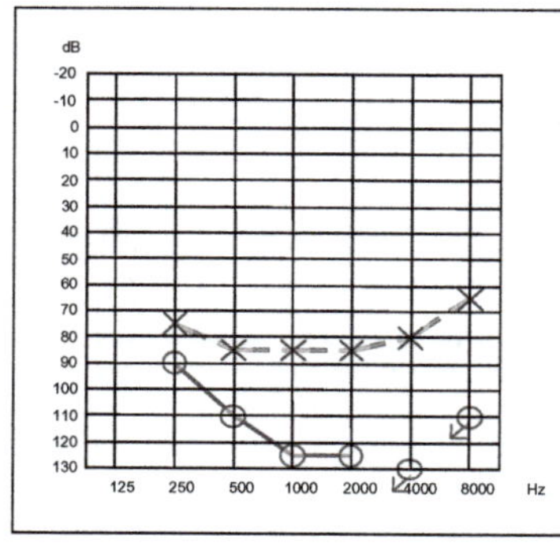

b) Postoperative, unaided

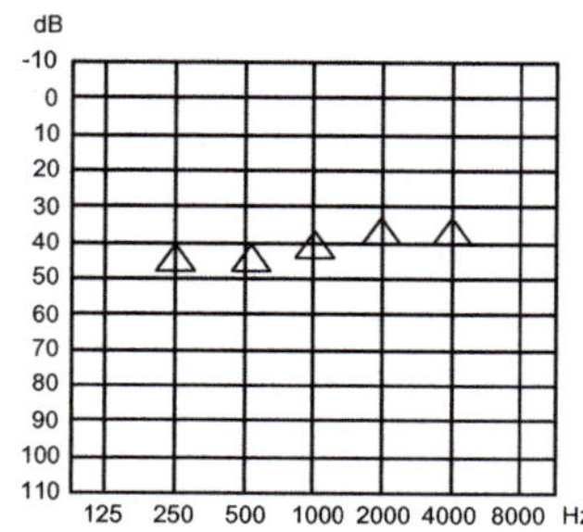

c) Postoperative, cochlear implant

Fig. 2. Case 2

hearing aid and preferred the sole use of the cochlear implant rather than the bimodal wearing of a hearing aid in the other side from her implanted ear.

Although total language development was delayed, as was anticipated from the delayed identification of her hearing loss, improvements were gradually observed, and her vocabulary also increased (Fig. 2b). In a series of Kyoto developmental tests [9] conducted in 2006, marked progress was observed, especially in language quotient (Fig. 2a). The patient is currently enrolled in a regular kindergarten and receives language training twice weekly.

Discussion

Some of the previous reports demonstrated poor language development after cochlear implant [11,12], while many others demonstrated preferable postoperative outcomes in the cases with AN/AD [13–18]. In each case presented here, cochlear implants were effective and greatly contributed to language development. Further investigation on a wider range of patients is necessary to determine whether cochlear implants are effective in all cases of AN/AD. However, at the very least, these findings suggest that cochlear implantation is a viable option in cases in which the possibility of AN/AD cannot be excluded.

Acknowledgments We deeply appreciate the patients and their families for their continuous cooperation in this study. This work is partly supported by the grant from the Ministry of Health, Labor and Welfare and the Ministry of Education, Science and Sports.

References

1. Hall JW III, Baer JE, Chase PA, et al (1994) Clinical application of otoacoustic emissions: what do we know about factors influencing measurement and analysis? Otolaryngol Head Neck Surg 110:22–38
2. Chiong CM, Dv Llanes EG, Tirona-Remulla AN, et al (2003) Neonatal hearing screening in a neonatal intensive care unit using distortion-product otoacoustic emissions. Acta Otolaryngol 123:215–218
3. Shivashankar N, Satishchandra P, Shashikala HR, et al (2003) Primary auditory neuropathy: an enigma. Acta Neurol Scand 108:130–135
4. Lopez-Diaz-de-Leon E, Silva-Rojas A, Ysunza A, et al (2003) Auditory neuropathy in Friedreich ataxia. A report of two cases. Int J Pediatr Otorhinolaryngol 67:641–648
5. Berlin CI, Hood L, Morlet T, et al (2003) Auditory neuropathy/dys-synchrony: diagnosis and management. Ment Retard Dev Disabil Res Rev 9:225–231
6. Ngo RY, Tan HK, Balakrishnan A, et al (2006) Auditory neuropathy/auditory dys-synchrony detected by universal newborn hearing screening. Int J Pediatr Otorhinolaryngol 70: 1299–1306
7. Berg AL, Spitzer JB, Towers HM, et al (2005) Newborn hearing screening in the NICU: profile of failed auditory brainstem response/passed otoacoustic emission. Pediatrics 116: 933–938
8. Fukuda S, Fukushima K, Toida N, et al (2003) Monosyllable speech perception of Japanese hearing aid users with prelingual hearing loss: implications for surgical indication of cochlear implant. Int J Pediatr Otorhinolaryngol 67:1061–1067
9. Fukushima K, Sugata K, Kasai N, et al (2002) Better speech performance in cochlear implant patients with GJB2-related deafness. Int J Pediatr Otorhinolaryngol 62:151–157
10. Kunisue K, Fukushima K, Nagayasu R, et al (2006) Longitudinal formant analysis after cochlear implantation in school-aged children. Int J Pediatr Otorhinolaryngol 70: 2033–2042
11. Miyamoto RT, Kirk KI, Renshaw J, et al (1999) Cochlear implantation in auditory neuropathy. Laryngoscope 109:181–185
12. Trautwein PG, Sininger YS, Nelson R (2000) Cochlear implantation of auditory neuropathy. J Am Acad Audiol 11:309–315
13. Shallop JK, Peterson A, Facer GW, et al (2001) Cochlear implants in five cases of auditory neuropathy: postoperative findings and progress. Laryngoscope 111:555–562
14. Buss E, Labadie RF, Brown CJ, et al (2002) Outcome of cochlear implantation in pediatric auditory neuropathy. Otol Neurotol 23:328–332
15. Madden C, Hilbert L, Rutter M, et al (2002) Pediatric cochlear implantation in auditory neuropathy Otol Neurotol 23:163–168
16. Mason JC, De Michele A, Stevens C, et al (2003) Cochlear implantation in patients with auditory neuropathy of varied etiologies. Laryngoscope 113:45–49
17. Peterson A, Shallop J, Driscoll C, et al (2003) Outcomes of cochlear implantation in children with auditory neuropathy. J Am Acad Audiol 14:188–201
18. Rouillon I, Marcolla A, Roux I, et al (2006) Results of cochlear implantation in two children with mutations in the OTOF gene. Int J Pediatr Otorhinolaryngol 70:689–696

Cochlear Implantation for a Child with Auditory Nerve Disease: a Case Report

Yukiko Shinjo, Yulian Jin, and Kimitaka Kaga

Summary

We present the case of a 5-year-old pediatric patient. On his first hospital visit at the age of 12 months, the results of his conditioned orientation response audiometry (COR) showed 30–45 dB HL, but his auditory brainstem responses (ABR) were bilaterally absent. However, the results of his distortion product otoacoustic emissions (DPOAE) test showed normal responses from both ears. Although he was fitted with hearing aids, he was still unable to show awareness of his parents' voice at normal loudness level. Because he was unable to speak any meaningful words up to the age of 3 years, he was implanted with a Nucleus CI 24 M device on the right ear when he was 3 years old. After the cochlear implantation, his auditory responses were better than before in home and school environments. His hearing threshold levels with the cochlear implant (CI) became stable and approximately 40 dB HL at all frequencies. His vocabulary and communication's skills have been gradually increasing up to now. Our patient shows that cochlear implantation can be effective for certain children with auditory nerve disease.

Key words Cochlear implantation, Auditory nerve disease, Auditory neuropathy, Infant, Hearing impairment

Introduction

Conventional hearing aids are rarely effective in patients with auditory nerve disease [1] or auditory neuropathy [2], which makes intervention and auditory habilitation difficult, particularly in infant patients. On the other hand, the efficacy of cochlear implantation in patients with auditory nerve disease is still uncertain.

National Institute of Sensory Organs, National Tokyo Medical Center, 2-5-1 Higashigaoka, Meguro-ku, Tokyo 152-8902, Japan

doi: 10.1007/978-4-431-09433-3_9, © Springer 2009

The following case presentation details the cochlear implantation of a pediatric patient with auditory nerve disease.

Case Report

We present the case of a 5-year-old pediatric patient. He was admitted to a hospital at the age of 12 months because of his inability to hear sound. His mother's pregnancy was normal, and his family history was negative for hearing impairment. He had no other significant medical history. His development of postural control and locomotion had been slightly delayed, and he began to walk by himself at the age of 18 months.

Auditory and Vestibular Examinations

On his first visit, the results of his conditioned orientation response audiometry (COR) showed 30–45 dB HL hearing threshold levels, but his auditory brainstem responses (ABR) were bilaterally absent. The results of his distortion product otoacoustic emissions (DPOAE) test showed normal responses from both ears (Fig. 1).

He also underwent routine vestibular examination. The ice water caloric test revealed no response bilaterally, but a rotational chair test showed normal results. Results of his vestibular-evoked myogenic potentials (VEMPs) test showed a small response on the left side, whereas it was normal on the right side (Fig. 2). The high-resolution temporal bone computed tomography (CT) scan and magnetic resonance imaging (MRI) revealed no abnormality in either ear.

He underwent COR repeatedly, but the results were different each time, so his hearing threshold levels were difficult to determine. He had worn hearing aids in both ears since the age of 18 months, but he did not like to wear the hearing aids and could not wear them for a long time. While wearing the hearing aids, he could be aware of loud sound, but could not be aware of his parents' voice at normal loudness level. He could say "ma-ma" or "pa-pa," but he was not able to speak any other meaningful words until he was 3 years old.

Cochlear Implantation

He was implanted with a Nucleus CI 24 M device on the right ear at the age of 3 years. The surgery proceeded successfully with no complications, with the full insertion of the device. We performed intraoperative measurement of electrically evoked compound action potentials (EAPs) using the Neural Response Telemetry System (NRT), and representative EAPs were recorded at every even electrode.

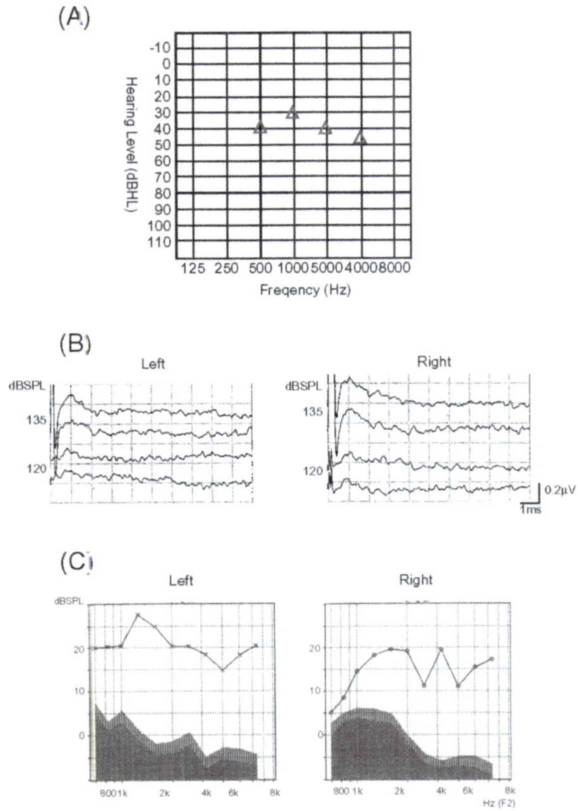

Fig. 1. Auditory examinations at the age of 12 months. **A** Results of the conditioned orientation response audiometry (COR) showed 30–45 dB HL hearing threshold levels. **B** The auditory brainstem responses (ABR) were absent on both sides at 135 dB SPL. **C** The results of the distortion product otoacoustic emissions (DPOAE) test showed normal responses from both ears

After the operation, the DPOAE response of the operated (right) side diminished, but that of the opposite (left) side did not change (Fig. 3).

He did not resist wearing the cochlear implant (CI), and he could wear it throughout the day only a week after the first sound stimulation. After 2 months, his auditory responses were better than before in home and school environments, and he was aware of faint sounds that he could not recognize before. After 5 months, he began to repeat the words of his parents or teachers.

At the age of 4 years and 8 months, the device broke down, so he underwent reimplantation with another device on the same side. The second operation also proceeded successfully, and his hearing ability has been maintained similar to that before the second operation. At present, the hearing threshold levels of the CI are stable and approximately 40 dB HL at all frequencies. The vowel recognition score became 100% without lip reading. His vocabulary is yet immature, but he can utter some words with actions. A spectrogram analysis of his voice revealed the differentiation of the characteristic formant of vowel sounds (Fig. 3).

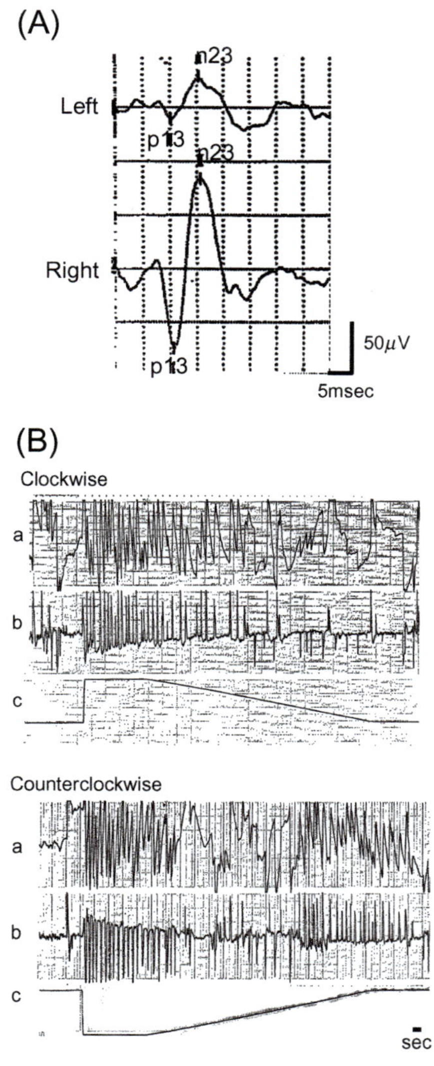

Fig. 2. Vestibular examinations. **A** Vestibular-evoked myogenic potential (VEMP) results. A small response was observed on the left side, whereas it was normal on the right side. **B** Rotational chair test results. Normal responses were observed on both sides. *a*, Angular displacement of eyes; *b*, rotational velocity of eyes; *c*, angular velocity of chair rotating

Discussion

The current broad definition of the term "auditory nerve disease" lumps together heterogeneous patients with a wide range of auditory dysfunctions, test results, and underlying etiologies. The site of lesion is difficult to determine. The presence of otoacoustic emissions and cochlear microphonics indicates that the outer hair cells are functioning, and the abnormal ABR indicates dysfunction of the peripheral portion of the auditory nerve. The symptoms pinpoint the area of disturbance to

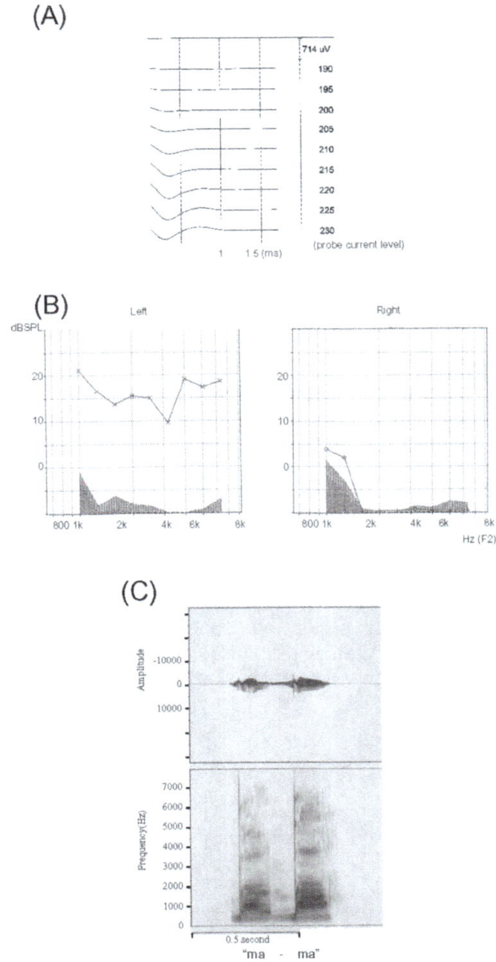

Fig. 3. **A** Intraoperative measurement of electrically evoked compound action potentials (EAPs) using the Neural Response Telemetry System (NRT). These results were normal at every even electrode. These representative EAPs were recorded from the no. 18 electrode. **B** DPOAE after the implantation. The DPOAE response of the cochlear implant (CI, right) side diminished, but that of the opposite (left) side did not change. **C** Spectrogram analysis of his voice saying "ma-ma" at the age of 5 years. Differentiation of the characteristic formant of vowel sounds was recognized

either the inner hair cells (IHCs), the synaptic junction between the IHCs and the auditory nerve, spiral ganglion neurons, or the peripheral portion of the auditory nerve.

The efficacy of cochlear implantation in patients with auditory nerve disease is still uncertain. Although initial reports of cochlear implantation in patients with auditory nerve disease and with Friedreich's ataxia recommended caution [3], more recent studies of children with only auditory nerve disease have demonstrated the benefit of cochlear implantation [4–6]. Our patient further shows that cochlear implantation can be effective for certain children with auditory nerve disease.

In most of these children with good outcomes of CI, the electrical EAPs showed normal responses. CI allows the opportunity to provide a supraphysiological electrical stimulation to the auditory nerve, and to reintroduce synchronous neural activity. These results suggest that the site of lesion in these patients may be the area from the IHCs to the spiral ganglions, and that some degree of function of the auditory nerve remains.

We conclude that CI can be successful for some patients with auditory nerve disease, and that the result of intraoperative electrical EAPs may reveal the outcome of CI. Auditory nerve disease should not be considered a contraindication to cochlear implantation.

References

1. Kaga K, Nakamura M, Shinogami M, et al (1996) Auditory nerve disease of both ears revealed by auditory brainstem responses, electrocochleography and otoacoustic emissions. Scand Audiol 25:233–238
2. Starr A, Picton TW, Sininger Y, et al (1996) Auditory neuropathy. Brain 119:741–753
3. Miyamoto RT, Kirk KI, Renshaw J, et al (1999) Cochlear implantation in auditory neuropathy. Laryngoscope 109:181–185
4. Trautwein PG, Sininger YS, Nelson R (2000) Cochlear implantation of auditory neuropathy. J Am Acad Audiol 11:309–315
5. Shallop JK, Peterson A, Facer GW, et al (2001) Cochlear implants in five cases of auditory neuropathy: postoperative findings and progress. Laryngoscope 111:555–562
6. Peterson A, Shallop J, Driscoll C, et al (2003) Outcomes of cochlear implantation in children with auditory neuropathy. J Am Acad Audiol 14:188–201

Part IV
Vestibular Neuropathy

Vestibular Neuropathy and Vestibular Evoked Myogenic Potential

Toshihisa Murofushi

Summary

"Vestibular neuropathy" is a new clinical entity, which could be defined as unilateral or bilateral dysfunction of the vestibular nerve. Vestibulopathy is a similar entity, although vestibulopathy includes dysfunction of the vestibular end-organs as well as the vestibular nerve. In this chapter, VEMP (vestibular evoked myogenic potentials) of idiopathic bilateral vestibulopathy (IBV) are first presented, and then the relationship between IBV and "vestibular and auditory neuropathy" is discussed. Seventeen patients diagnosed as IBV were enrolled. Diagnostic criteria were as follows: (1) bilaterally decreased caloric responses (maximum slow phase eye velocity ≤10°/s), (2) no associated hearing loss, and (3) exclusion of bilateral vestibular dysfunction from known causes and familial cases. Patient age ranged from 33 to 75 years. Acoustic VEMP were bilaterally absent in 6 patients, unilaterally absent in 6 patients, unilaterally decreased in 2 patients, and normal in 3 patients. Combined application of galvanic VEMP suggested that the lesion site should be mainly in the vestibular nerve. Some patients with IBV had prolonged interpeak intervals between waves I and III of ABR. In conclusion, (1) IBV could be vestibular neuropathy, and (2) there could be overlapping between vestibular neuropathy and auditory neuropathy in adult cases.

Key words Idiopathic bilateral vestibulopathy, Vestibular neuritis, Inferior vestibular nerve, Vestibular evoked myogenic potential, Saccule

---

Department of Otolaryngology, Teikyo University School of Midicine Mizonokuchi Hospital, 3-8-3 Mizonokuchi, Takatsu-ku, Kawasaki 213-8507, Japan

doi: 10.1007/978-4-431-09433-3_10,

Introduction

"Vestibular neuropathy" is not a common clinical entity. It could be defined as unilateral or bilateral dysfunction of the vestibular nerve. Vestibulopathy is a similar entity to vestibular neuropathy, although vestibulopathy includes dysfunction of the vestibular labyrinth as well as the vestibular nerve. Idiopathic bilateral vestibulopathy (IBV) is a clinical entity proposed by Baloh et al. [1]. IBV represents bilateral dysfunction of the peripheral vestibular system resulting from unknown causes.

Vestibular evoked myogenic potential (VEMP) is a kind of evoked electromyography (EMG) [2,3]. Originally, VEMP was recorded on the sternocleidomastoid muscle (SCM) as responses to relatively intense click stimulation [2,3]. VEMP has been regarded as a vestibulo(sacculo)-collic reflex and applied as a clinical test of the vestibular system. Although VEMP findings in various diseases have been reported [2–11], only limited information is available concerning VEMP in IBV [12,13]. In this chapter, I first cover VEMP of IBV and then discuss the association of IBV with vestibular neuropathy.

Materials and Methods

Subjects

Seventeen patients (10 men and 7 women, 33–75 years of age, mean, 59 years of age) diagnosed as having IBV were enrolled into this study. The age distribution of patients is shown in Fig. 1.

Diagnostic criteria of IBV were as follows.

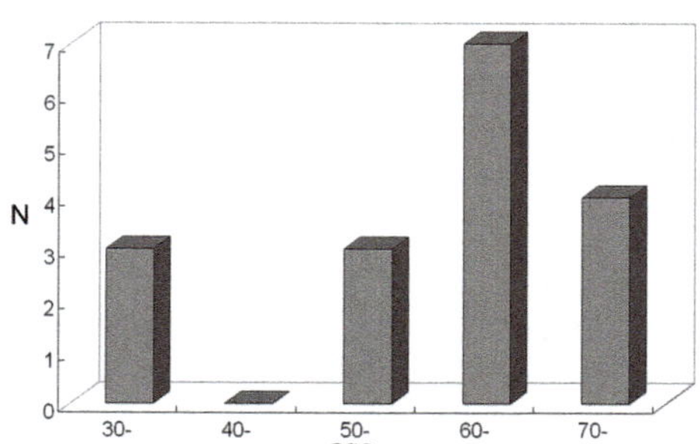

Fig. 1. Age distribution of patients with idiopathic bilateral vestibulopathy (IBV)

1. Bilateral decreased caloric responses (maximum slow phase eye velocity: 10°/s or slower in the caloric test using ice water).
2. No associated hearing loss.
3. Exclusion of bilateral vestibular dysfunction by known causes such as meningitis or aminoglycoside ototoxicity.
4. Exclusion of familial cases.

Informed consent was obtained from each subject according to the Declaration of Helsinki. Ethical approval was received from the local ethics committee.

Methods

Subjects underwent medical history taking, pure tone audiometry, VEMP testing to clicks, and caloric testing. Some subjects also underwent ABR (auditory brainstem responses) and VEMP testing to galvanic stimulation [14,15].

For recording VEMP, active recording electrodes were placed on the middle of the SCM while inactive electrodes were on the lateral end of the upper sternum. The ground electrode was on the nasion. Clicks (95 dB nHL, 0.1 ms) were presented to all the subjects. Electromyographic (EMG) activities were amplified and bandpass filtered (20–2000 Hz). The stimulation rate was 5 Hz, and the analysis window was 50 ms. The responses to 100 stimuli were averaged twice with the contraction of the SCM by raising the head from a pillow in the supine position.

To compare the amplitude of p13-n23 of VEMP responses on the affected side with those on the unaffected side, the percent VEMP asymmetry (percent VA) of each patient was calculated as 100(Au – Aa)/(Aa + Au), where Au is the p13-n23 amplitude on the unaffected side and Aa is the p13-n23 amplitude on the affected side [4]. On the basis of the results from normal subjects, the normal range of the percent VA was placed at –34.1 to 34.1 (within mean + 2 SD) [4].

For galvanic VEMP, 3 mA (1 ms) currents were used. The electrodes for stimulation were placed on the mastoid (cathode) and the forehead (anode). The responses to 50 stimuli were averaged twice with the contraction of the SCM by raising the head from a pillow in the supine position. To remove artifacts of galvanic stimuli, we subtracted the responses obtained without SCM contraction from the responses with SCM contraction [15]. Other methods for recording galvanic VEMP were the same as those of VEMP to clicks.

To record ABRs, surface electrodes were placed on the ipsilateral mastoid and the vertex. An electrode on the nasion served as the ground. Signals at the vertex to the ipsilateral mastoid were amplified and bandpass filtered (100–3000 Hz). Clicks (0.1 ms, 85 dB nHL) were presented at the rate of 10 Hz, and the analysis window was 10 ms. The responses to 1000 stimuli were averaged twice.

All the subjects also underwent caloric tests. The caloric nystagmus was recorded using electronystagmography (ENG).

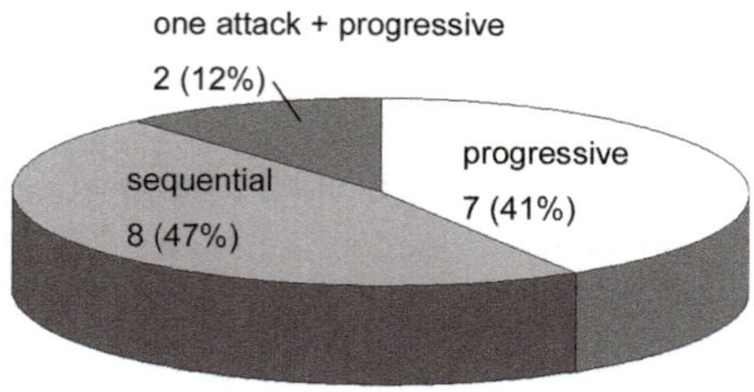

Fig. 2. Classification of patients according to types of clinical course

Results

Classification by Clinical Course

According to the clinical course, patients were classified into three types: (1) progressive type (7 patients), sequential type (8 patients), and one attack and progressive type (2 patients) (Fig. 2).

Before presenting test results, typical patients of each type are described.

Patient 1 (Progressive Type)

A 36-year-old man came to our clinic with a complaint of disequilibrium beginning 1 year earlier. He did not note hearing loss or rotatory vertigo. His medical history was unremarkable. On examination, he had no gaze, positional, or positioning nystagmus. His equilibrium became worse with eyes closed. In caloric testing (ice water), the maximum slow phase eye velocities were 4°/s on the left and 5°/s on the right. VEMPs were normal on both sides (Fig. 3). His pure tone hearing was normal.

Patient 2 (Sequential Type)

A 75-year-old woman came to our clinic with a complaint of disequilibrium since the last vertigo attack that had occurred 2 months earlier. She had experienced three episodes of rotatory vertigo. Her medical history was unremarkable. On examination, she showed symmetrical high tone sensorineural hearing loss, probably a result of aging. She had no gaze, positional, or positioning nystagmus. Her equilibrium was unstable even with eyes open and became worse with eyes closed. In caloric testing (ice water), the maximum slow phase eye velocities were 0°/s on the left and 1°/s on the right. VEMPs were absent on the left but present on the right (Fig. 4).

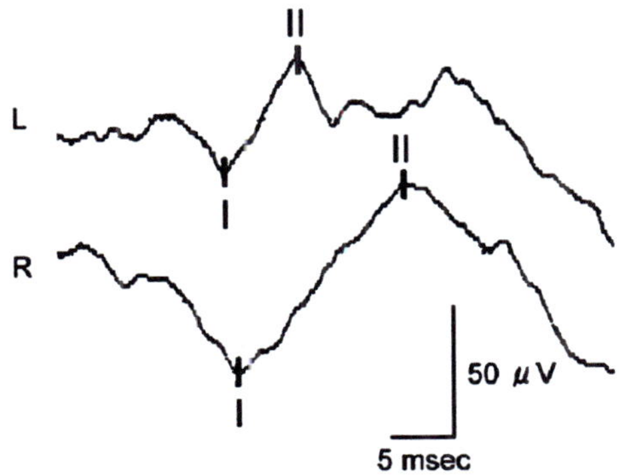

Fig. 3. Vestibular evoked myogenic potentials (VEMP) of a 36-year-old man with IBV (progressive type). He showed normal responses on both sides

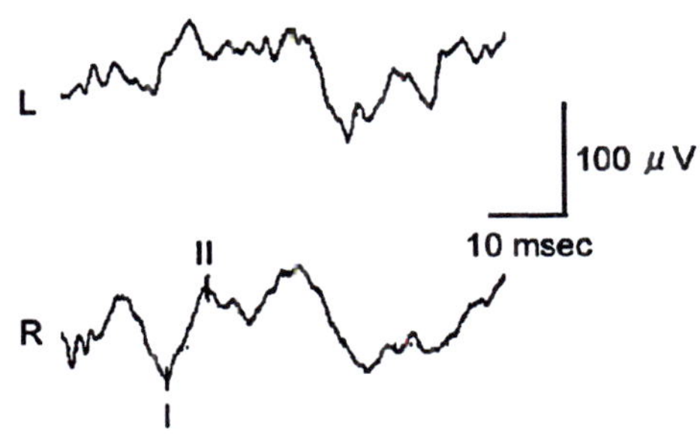

Fig. 4. VEMP of a 75-year-old woman with IBV (sequential type). Her VEMPs were normal on the right but absent on the left

Patient 3 (One Attack and Progressive Type)

A 53-year-old woman came to our clinic with a complaint of disequilibrium and oscillopsia during walking beginning 5 years earlier. She had experienced one episode of severe rotatory vertigo 15 years before. Then, she was diagnosed as having left vestibular neuritis. She had undergone medical treatment for chronic hepatitis. On examination, her pure tone hearing was normal. She had no gaze, positional, or positioning nystagmus. Her equilibrium was unstable with eyes closed. In caloric testing (ice water), the maximum slow phase eye velocities were 0°g/s on the left and 10°/s on the right. VEMPs were normal on the left but absent on the right.

Table 1. Clinical course of idiopathic bilateral vestibulopathy (IBV) and vestibular evoked myogenic potentials (VEMP) results

	Progressive type	Sequential type	One attack + progressive type
Bilaterally absent	3	3	0
Unilaterally absent	2	3	1
Unilaterally decreased	0	1	1
Bilaterally normal	2	1	0

Data are numbers of patients

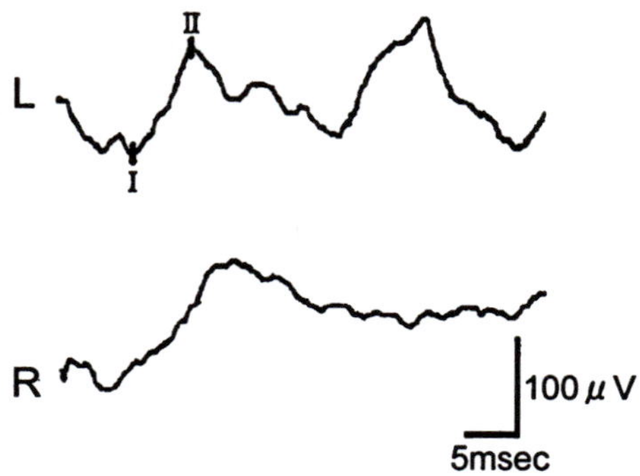

Fig. 5. Galvanic VEMP of a 75-year-old man with IBV (progressive type). His VEMPs to acoustic stimuli were absent on the right, and his galvanic VEMPs were also absent on the right

VEMP

Click VEMPs were bilaterally absent in 6 patients, unilaterally absent in 6 patients, unilaterally decreased in 2 patients, and bilaterally normal in 3 patients. Twenty of the 34 sides (58%) showed abnormal VEMPs, which means that 14 of the 17 patients (82%) had abnormal VEMP results.

There was no significant relationship between VEMP results and types of clinical course (Table 1) ($P = 0.5$, χ^2 test).

Galvanic VEMPs were applied to three patients. Among the six sides, four sides of the three patients showed absent galvanic VEMPs. When a side showed absence of VEMP to acoustic stimulation, it also showed absence of galvanic VEMP (Fig. 5).

Caloric Tests

Caloric responses to ice water were bilaterally absent in 4 patients, unilaterally absent and unilaterally decreased in 4 patients, and bilaterally decreased in 9 patients.

ABR

ABRs were recorded in four patients. Two sides of the two patients showed slightly prolonged interpeak intervals between waves I and III (2.54 and 2.46 ms; normal range, 2.0–2.4 ms).

Discussion

It is not easy to differentiate vestibular nerve lesions from labyrinthine lesions in patients with peripheral vestibular dysfunction. Murofushi et al. [15] reported that the combined application of galvanic VEMP in a patient with absent acoustic VEMP was useful for the differential diagnosis of labyrinthine lesions from retro-labyrinthine ones. They reported that patients with labyrinthine lesions, such as Meniere's disease, showed normal galvanic VEMP despite absent responses to clicks, but patients with nerve lesions, such as acoustic neuroma, showed absent or decreased responses to galvanic stimuli, as well as click. This method has been applied to other types of vestibular disorders [16,17]. This combined application to patients with IBV suggested that the principal lesion site of IBV could be in the vestibular nerve, although the number of patients was still small. In other words, IBV could be idiopathic vestibular neuropathy.

Also, the present study showed that IBV could be divided into two groups; the abnormal VEMP group and the normal VEMP group. The former has lesions not only in the superior vestibular nerve but also in the inferior vestibular nerve [3]. The latter has lesions in the superior vestibular nerve but spared functions in the inferior vestibular nerve. If decreased responses in the caloric test had not been included in the diagnostic criteria of IBV, some patients with IBV could have shown normal caloric responses but abnormal VEMPs [18]. Then, IBV could be classified into three groups: superior vestibular neuropathy, inferior vestibular neuropathy, and superior/inferior vestibular neuropathy.

We are also interested in the relationship between auditory neuropathy and vestibular neuropathy. Sheykholeslami et al. [19] reported that 3 adult patients with auditory neuropathy (auditory nerve disease) [20,21] had vestibular hypo-function; absent VEMP and decreased caloric responses. Fujikawa and Starr [22] reported that 9 of the 14 patients with auditory neuropathy had abnormal caloric responses. These findings suggested that patients with auditory neuropathy could also have vestibular neuropathy. On the other hand, among the 17 patients in this study, 2 patients had slightly prolonged interpeak interval between waves I and III in ABR testing. This finding suggested that patients with IBV might have damage in the cochlear nerve. Therefore, auditory (cochlear) neuropathy and vestibular neuropathy might be a part of a larger clinical entity, neuropathy of the eighth cranial nerve.

References

1. Baloh RW, Jacobson K, Honrubia V (1989) Idiopathic bilateral vestibulopathy. Neurology 39:272–275
2. Colebatch JG, Halmagyi GM, Skuse NF (1994) Myogenic potentials generated by a click-evoked vestibulocollic reflex. J Neurol Neurosurg Psychiatry 57:190–197
3. Murofushi T, Halmagyi GM, Yavor RA, et al (1996) Absent vestibular evoked myogenic potentials in vestibular neurolabyrinthitis: an indicator of inferior vestibular nerve involvement? Arch Otolaryngol Head Neck Surg 122:845–848
4. Murofushi T, Matsuzaki M, Mizuno M (1998) Vestibular evoked myogenic potentials in patients with acoustic neuromas. Arch Otolaryngol Head Neck Surg 124:509–512
5. Patko T, Vidal PP, Vibert N, et al (2003) Vestibular evoked myogenic potentials in patients suffering from an unilateral acoustic neuroma: a study of 170 patients. Clin Neurophysiol 114:1344–1350
6. Rauch SD, Zhou G, Kujuwa SG, et al (2004) Vestibular evoked myogenic potentials show altered tuning in patients with Meniere's disease. Otol Neurotol 25:333–338
7. Ohki M, Matsuzaki M, Sugasawa K, et al (2002) Vestibular evoked myogenic potentials with contralateral delayed endolymphatic hydrops. Eur Arch Otorhinolaryngol 259:24–26
8. Ohki M, Matsuzaki M, Sugasawa K, et al (2002) Vestibular evoked myogenic potentials in ipsilateral delayed endolymphatic hydrops. ORL (Basel) 64:424–428
9. Iwasaki S, Takai Y, Murofushi T (2005) Extent of lesions in idiopathic sudden hearing loss with vertigo: study using click and galvanic VEMP. Arch Otolaryngol Head Neck Surg 131:857–862
10. Ozeki H, Matsuzaki M, Murofushi T (1999) Vestibular evoked myogenic potentials in three patients with bilateral profound hearing loss. ORL (Basel) 61:80–83
11. Brantberg K, Bergenius J, Tribukait A (1999) Vestibular-evoked myogenic potentials in patients with dehiscence of the superior semicircular canal. Acta Otolaryngol (Stockh) 119:633–640
12. Matsuzaki M, Murofushi T (2001) Vestibular evoked myogenic potentials in patients with idiopathic bilateral vestibulopathy. ORL (Basel) 63:349–352
13. Fujimoto C, Iwasaki S, Matsuzaki M, et al (2005) The site of lesion in idiopathic bilateral vestibulopathy: study by galvanic VEMP. Acta Otolaryngol 125:430–432
14. Watson SRD, Colebatch JG (1998) Vestibulocollic reflexes evoked by short-duration galvanic stimulation in man. J Physiol 513:587–597
15. Murofushi T, Takegoshi H, Ohki M, et al (2002) Galvanic-evoked myogenic responses in patients with an absence of click-evoked vestibulo-collic reflexes. Clin Neurophysiol 113:305–309
16. Murofushi T, Monobe H, Ozeki H, et al (2003) The site of lesions in "vestibular neuritis"; study by galvanic VEMP. Neurology 61:417–418
17. Ozeki H, Iwasaki S, Ushio M, et al (2006) The lesion site of vestibular dysfunction in Ramsay Hunt syndrome. J Vestib Res 16:217–222
18. Iwasaki S, Takai Y, Ito K, et al (2005) Abnormal vestibular evoked myogenic potentials in the presence of normal caloric responses. Otol Neurootol 26:1196–1199
19. Sheykholeslami K, Kaga K, Murofushi T, et al (2000) Vestibular function in auditory neuropathy. Acta Otolaryngol (Stockh) 120:849–854
20. Kaga K, Nakamura M, Shinogami M, et al (1996) Auditory nerve disease of both ears revealed by auditory brainstem responses, electrocochleography and otoacoustic emissions. Scand Audiol 25:233–238
21. Starr A, Picton TW, Sininger Y, et al (1996) Auditory neuropathy. Brain 119:741–753
22. Fujikawa S, Starr A (2000) Vestibular neuropathy accompanying auditory and peripheral neuropathies. Arch Otolaryngol Head Neck Surg 126:1453–1456

Impulsive Testing of Semicircular Canal Function

G. Michael Halmagyi, Konrad P. Weber, Swee T. Aw, Michael J. Todd, and Ian S. Curthoys

Summary

Head impulses are brisk, passive, unpredictable rotations of the head in the plane of parallel semicircular canal pairs. In a normal test, the vestibulo-ocular reflex stabilizes gaze in space by compensating head rotations with equal eye rotations to the opposite direction. In a patient with impaired semicircular canal function, the eyes move with the head, and the patient needs to make a catch-up saccade back to the target. Three-dimensional measurement of eye movement responses to head impulses in individual semicircular canal planes allows determining the gain of the angular vestibulo-ocular reflex in each of the six canals. At the bedside, the head impulse test is an easy way for the clinician to identify unilateral or bilateral impairment of semicircular canal function; it identifies the catch-up saccades back to the target after head rotation as an indirect sign of peripheral vestibular loss. In patients with acute spontaneous vertigo, the head impulse test helps to distinguish between a peripheral vestibular loss, where the test is positive, and a central vestibular lesion, where the test is usually negative.

Key words Head impulse, Vestibulo-ocular reflex, Catch-up saccade, Semicircular canal, Eye movements

Background

The semicircular canals (SCCs) operate as push-pull pairs by means of the bidirectional morphological and physiological polarization of the hair cell bundles on the cupula [1]. During any head rotation, displacement of the hair cells towards the kinocilium depolarizes hair cells and generates excitation, while displacement away

Neurology Department, Royal Prince Alfred Hospital, Camperdown, Sydney, NSW 2050, Australia

doi: 10.1007/978-4-431-09433-3_11,

from the kinocilium hyperpolarizes hair cells and generates inhibition. In response to a head rotation such as a head impulse, one SCC of the push-pull pair is excited while the other is inhibited, generating the total angular vestibulo-ocular reflex (VOR) from direct excitation and indirect disinhibition. In the lateral (horizontal) SCC, ampullopetal endolymph flow causes excitation whereas ampullofugal flow causes inhibition. However, for the vertical SCCs, that is, the anterior (superior) and posterior SCCs, ampullofugal flow causes excitation and ampullopetal flow causes inhibition. It is this directional polarization, which produces the on-off directional asymmetry of the VOR generated by a single SCC, that is summarized in Ewald's second law [2,3] and is the key to diagnosing disorders of individual SCC function.

The eye movement response to a head impulse depends on the VOR and can be used as a quick, reliable, bedside screening test of SCC function with no equipment needed [4]. In the clinical head impulse test of normal subjects, the clinician sees (almost) nothing: during and after a rapid head rotation the subject is continuously looking at the fixation target. A patient with impaired SCC function, however, cannot keep looking at the fixation target during the head impulse and needs to make a catch-up saccade, easily detected by the clinician, to refixate the target. The laboratory method does require sophisticated equipment, but provides precise information about three-dimensional eye movements from which one can infer the function of individual SCC. The head impulse test complements the other standard vestibular function tests, because in contrast to the caloric test, for example, it measures the VOR with a physiological stimulus and can independently evaluate individual function of each of the six SCC in three dimensions.

Definitions

A head impulse consists of a single, brisk head rotation of 20°–30° amplitude, approximately in the plane of a SCC pair. The subject's task is to focus on a fixation target. Head impulses can be generated in four different ways:

1. Passive head-only impulses, in which the clinician grasps and rotates the patient's head [3–10].
2. Active head-only impulses, in which patients themselves rotate their own head [11,12].
3. Passive head-only impulses with some electromechanical device rotating only the head [13–15].
4. Passive whole-body impulses with some electromechanical device rotating the whole body [16–18].

Passive head impulses are useful at the bedside because no equipment is needed. For recording purposes, a feedback signal for the examiner allows to deliver standardized head impulses [12]. Compared to passive head impulses, active head impulses turned out to be unhelpful for diagnosing a vestibular deficit [12]. In active head impulses, the measured VOR gain is higher, and catch-up saccades occur more frequently during rather than after head rotation, where they are imperceptible to a clinical observer. Passive head impulse testing with electromechanical devices to deliver standardized stimuli has been proven feasible but requires sophisticated equipment [13–15]. Passive whole-body impulses in a rotational chair exclude the possible influence of the cervico-ocular reflex but at the price of a limited angular acceleration [16–18].

Head impulses are usually applied in the plane of the parallel SCC pairs. Horizontal head impulses about the Z-axis excite the ipsilateral and inhibit the contralateral lateral canal (Fig. 1A). The vertical canal pairs can be individually tested along their approximate right-anterior and left-posterior (RALP) and left-anterior and right-posterior (LARP) planes to activate the respective anterior and posterior SCC pairs, as shown in Fig. 1B [8,10,19].

The terms yaw, pitch, roll, LARP, and RALP refer to head rotation directions defined with reference to the subject (see Fig. 1). According to convention, which follows the right-hand rule [20], left, down, and clockwise head or eye rotations are positive, while right, up, and counterclockwise directions are negative. Clockwise direction means that the upper pole of the head or eye is rotated towards the subject's right and counterclockwise direction means towards the subject's left.

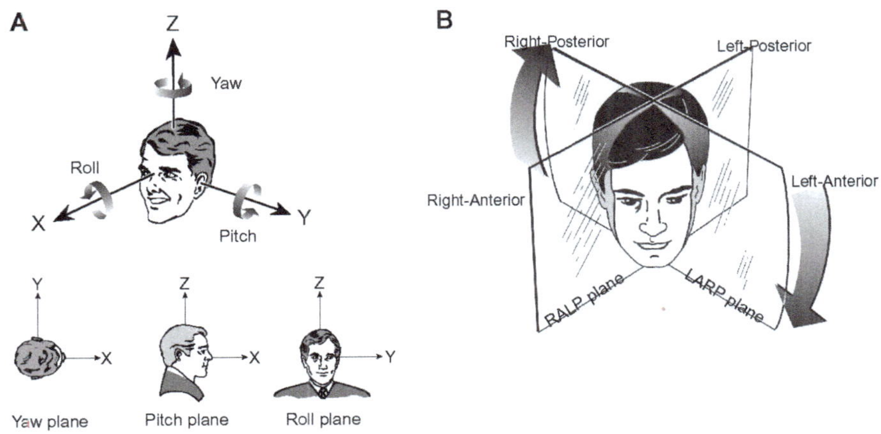

Fig. 1. **A** Head-fixed coordinate system obeying the right-hand rule used to express angular eye position and eye velocity vectors. Positive directions of eye rotations are designated by *arrow directions*. Yaw impulses are head rotations in the yaw plane about the Z-axis; pitch impulses are head rotations in the pitch plane about the *Y*-axis, and roll impulses are head rotation in the roll plane about the *X*-axis. **B** LARP (left anterior–right posterior canals) and RALP (right anterior–left posterior canals) impulses are head impulses in the *LARP and RALP planes*

Measuring the Impulsive VOR

Scleral Search Coil Method

The search coil technique [6,21–23] is the standard method used to measure the head impulse test either in two or three dimensions.

Head and eye positions can be recorded in two dimensions with single-search coils [3–5,24,25] or in three dimensions with dual-search coils [6–8,10,19,26].

The subject wears search coils monocular or binocular on the eyes to measure angular eye positions while another search coil is attached to a dental impression bite-bar to measure the angular head position. The dental impression bite-bar is recommended to prevent head coil slippage. The search coils are precalibrated before each recording. The subject is seated with the head in the center of the magnetic field coil system wearing the head and eye search coils. The magnetic field coil system is available in either the two-field or three-field configuration.

The rationale of in vitro calibration is to determine the gains and offsets of the signals from each search coil induced by the magnetic fields. All coils are simultaneously mounted on a Fick gimbal. When a two-field magnetic system is used, the gimbal is moved in yaw, pitch, or roll calibration positions between ±20° in steps of 5° and the gains and offsets for each search coil are determined. Maximum errors and cross-coupling are less than 2% [6].

When a three-field magnetic system is used, initially offset voltages from undesirable noise pickup and internal amplifier biases are compensated by placing the search coil in a soft iron tube, which isolates it from the magnetic fields, while the amplifier offsets are nulled [27]. Then, the annulus is placed on a gimbal system and rotated in six positions, each of which picks up the maximum voltage induced by one magnetic field in one search coil (two coils times three directions for each dual-search coil). These voltage signals are then used to compute the orientation of the dual search coil in the space-fixed magnetic frame.

To obtain good temporal resolution in the head impulse test, a sampling frequency of the search coil signals of at least 500 Hz is needed. The resolution of the ADC (analogue to digital converter) should be at least 16 bits so that digital head or eye velocity derived from its position signal has good signal-to-noise ratio.

Videooculographic Method

Although the search coil technique has fulfilled all the necessary criteria for quantification of the head impulse test, it is technically demanding and difficult to translate to a clinical setting. Unfortunately, the technology for videographic eye movement recording still has to overcome several limitations, hampering its use in the head impulse test. First, slippage of the head-fixed video camera during high acceleration head rotation may cause artifacts, which can be mistaken as a normal VOR response. Second, limited spatial and temporal resolution of the videographic recording system makes it difficult to calculate digital head and eye velocity to determine VOR gain from the head impulse test. No doubt, with technological improvement, it will soon become feasible to record high-quality head impulse responses with a video system.

Data Analysis

Head, gaze, and eye positions are analysed in three dimensions as rotation vectors [28,29] or Euler angles [29,30]. Head and gaze positions are the orientations of the head and eye in space-fixed coordinates. Eye position is the orientation of the eye in head-fixed coordinates [6]. Head, gaze and eye velocities are calculated from their respective positions [29]. A rotation of the coordinate reference frame by 45° about the yaw-axis allows reexpression of these vectors as rotations about the approximate preferred axis of individual vertical SCCs [8] and display of the angular VOR related to the anterior and posterior SCCs (see Fig. 1B).

The gain of the angular VOR in response to a head impulse should be analyzed in the first 70-ms period after impulse onset as catch-up saccades made during yaw impulses may have latencies as short as 70 ms [17,31]. Both the cervico-ocular reflex [32] and smooth pursuit [33] have latencies greater than 100 ms.

Vestibulo-Ocular Reflex Latency, Gain, Direction, and Symmetry

The latency of the VOR in response to head impulses has been estimated to be about 6–10 ms in humans [6,13,14] and also in animals [34,35]. In humans, one method of estimating latency is to shift the eye velocity at 1-ms intervals towards the head velocity, and the least-squares difference between the head and eye velocity is determined after each shift. The latency is the time interval shifted when the least-squares difference between the head and eye velocity is minimum [6]. Another method is to measure the time interval between the intersections of the linear regressions of (or least square fit) head and eye velocities with the time axis [14].

VOR gain can be described in at least four different ways:

1. Velocity gain in one dimension, referenced to the orthogonal yaw, pitch, and roll axes [6,7,9] or to the rotated reference frames of LARP and RALP axes [8,19], calculated as instantaneous eye velocity divided by head velocity, at or close to peak head velocity [6,7,10,14].

2. Acceleration gain, calculated as the ratio between the slopes of eye and head velocities for a period before peak head velocity [14,26,31].

3. Three-dimensional speed gain, defined as the ratio of eye velocity magnitude (eye speed) to head velocity magnitude (head speed), measures the total angular VOR in response to head rotations about a single axis, i.e., yaw, pitch, or roll [6].

4. Impulsive canal paresis, described as three-dimensional gaze instability during a head impulse and defined as the ratio of gaze velocity to head velocity in SCC coordinates [36,37]. Impulsive canal paresis is defined close to peak head velocity, in response to a head rotation towards the on-direction of a SCC, along its SCC plane [19]. Gaze and head velocities are normalized by dividing each velocity by the magnitude of peak head velocity in each trial, and then gaze and head velocities are determined in SCC coordinates.

Based on the VOR gain to each side (g_r, g_l), the percentage of VOR asymmetry (g_s) can be calculated as follows [13,31]:

$$g_s = \frac{g_r - g_l}{g_r + g_l} \times 100$$

The direction of the input-output kinematics of the VOR can be described as a misalignment angle, the instantaneous angle by which the eye rotation axis deviates from perfect alignment with the head rotation axis in three dimensions [6].

Impulsive Testing and Catch-Up Saccades

During head impulses, the VOR generates compensatory eye movements approximately equal in amplitude and in the opposite direction to stabilize the gaze in space (Fig. 2A,D). During rapid rotation toward the side of a peripheral vestibular lesion, the absence of angular VOR results in loss of normal compensatory eye movements, and the patient would make a catch-up saccade to refixate the target (Fig. 2B,E,C,F). Observation of these catch-up saccades forms the basis of a clinical judgment of individual SCC function at the bedside to assess angular vestibular deficits [4,38–40].

These catch-up saccades can be classified as overt or covert saccades (Fig. 2E,F) [31]. Covert saccades occur during head rotation (head velocity >0) and are imperceptible to a clinical observer. Overt saccades appear after head rotation and are detectable by the clinician. The percentage of head impulse trials with covert saccades and the amplitude of the consecutive overt saccades are useful parameters to judge whether a measured vestibular deficit can be detected at the bedside.

Finally, the contribution of both VOR and catch-up saccades on gaze stabilization during head impulses can be estimated graphically with a phase-plane analysis by plotting gaze velocity versus gaze position [41].

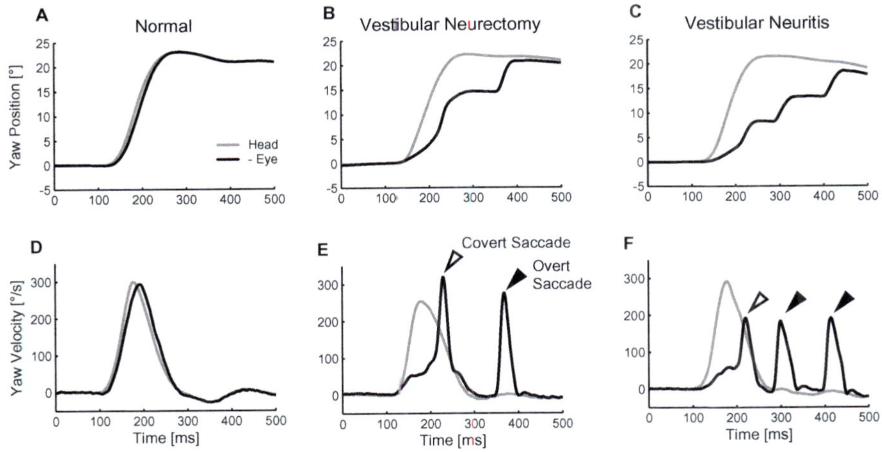

Fig. 2. Typical examples of eye movement responses to yaw head impulses from a healthy normal subject (**A, D**), a patient after left unilateral vestibular neurectomy (**B, E**), and a patient after left unilateral vestibular neuritis (**C, F**). Eye signals are inverted for ease of comparison with head signals. In the normal subject, the compensatory horizontal eye velocity to a yaw-left impulse is equal and opposite to head velocity and results in a stable gaze direction. The loss of left lateral canal function in both patients results in lower compensatory horizontal eye velocity than head velocity, and thus eye position errors occur. These patients have to generate catch-up saccades (*arrows*) to stabilize gaze direction. Overt catch-up saccades (*filled arrows*) after head rotation are detectable in bedside testing whereas covert saccades (*empty arrows*) during head rotation remain imperceptible to the clinical observer

Clinical Applications of Impulsive VOR Testing

Total Unilateral Vestibular Deafferentation

Typical examples of angular VOR in response to yaw, LARP, and RALP head impulses in a healthy subject and in a subject with total unilateral loss after unilateral vestibular deafferentation are displayed in Fig. 3. The head impulses are executed approximately in the plane of each individual SCC, so that the results can be displayed with reference to the lateral, anterior, and posterior canals on the left and right sides. All the eye signals are inverted for ease of comparison with the head signals.

In the healthy normal subject, the eye velocity is approximately equal and opposite to head velocity (Fig. 3A,C,E). The normal VOR gain in response to yaw impulses is ~1.0 in humans [3,5,6,8] and in animals [34,42]. The VOR gain of the diagonal LARP and RALP head impulses is ~0.7–0.8. Normal VOR gain of roll impulses is ~0.6–0.7 and that of pitch impulses is ~1.0 [6]. In the LARP and RALP directions, the head and eye velocity vectors are derived from the pitch and roll components, and hence the normal VOR gain of the diagonal

LARP and RALP head impulses is ~0.7–0.8 in humans [8,26] and in animals [35].

After unilateral vestibular deafferentation, the angular VOR in response to head impulses directed toward each of the three deafferented SCCs is consistently deficient. Figure 3 (B,D,F) shows head impulses directed toward each SCC in a representative unilateral vestibular deafferented subject following left vestibular neurectomy as treatment for a left vestibular schwannoma. The VOR gain during head impulses toward the lesioned left SCCs was low at ~0.2–0.3 in all three SCCs, but the responses toward the intact right side are close to normal limits (similar deficits are also recorded in animals) [34,35,42–44].

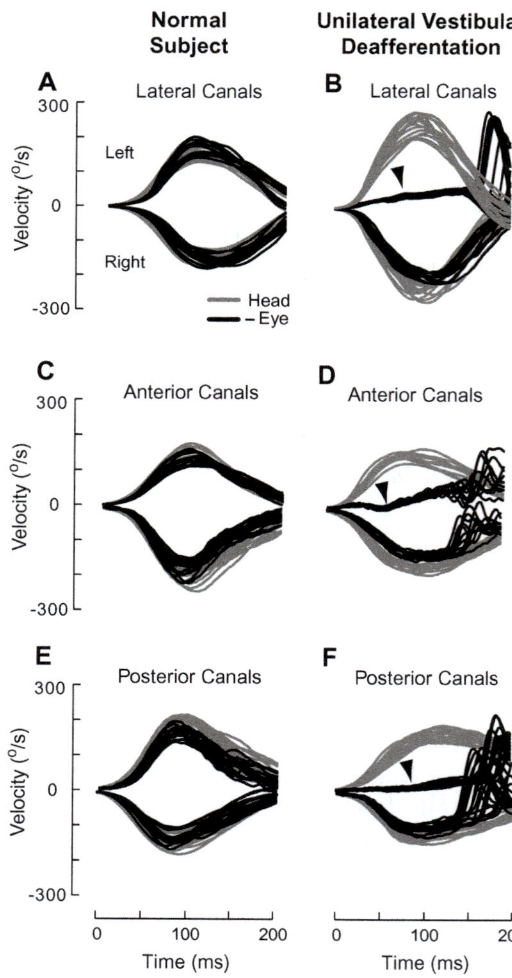

Fig. 3. Time series of multiple trials of yaw, LARP, and RALP head impulses directed approximately toward each individual semicircular canal in a healthy normal subject (*left column*) and in a unilateral vestibular deafferented patient (*right column*). Eye velocity has been inverted for ease of comparison with head velocity. **A, C, E** In the normal subject, eye velocity is approximately equal and opposite to head velocity for all six semicircular canals, reflecting a normal angular vestibulo-ocular reflex (VOR) and semicircular canal function. The VOR gains in the normal subject are lateral SCCs, ~1.0; and superior and posterior SCCs, ~0.9. **B, D, F** In the left unilateral vestibular deafferented patient, the angular VOR is deficient (*arrows*) in the left lateral, superior, and posterior canals with VOR gains of ~0.2–0.3, indicating total unilateral loss of function in these semicircular canals

Vestibular Neuritis

Vestibular neuritis is a common acute spontaneous unilateral peripheral vestibulopathy with a clinical syndrome that consists of vertigo, nystagmus, postural imbalance, nausea, and vomiting with preserved hearing and no evidence of brainstem dysfunction [9,19,45–48]. The extent of involvement of the vestibular nerve or the labyrinth by vestibular neuritis can be inferred from head impulse assessment of individual SCC function [19]. The superior vestibular nerve innervates the lateral and anterior SCCs, the utricle, and a part of the saccule, whereas the inferior vestibular nerve innervates the posterior SCC and most of the saccule. Because of the innervation pattern of the SCCs, complete functional losses from all three SCCs on one side suggest a complete vestibular neuritis involving both the superior and inferior vestibular nerves together (Fig. 4A,D,G). Functional losses from lateral and anterior canals suggest selective superior vestibular neuritis (Fig. 4B,E,H), whereas functional loss from the posterior canal alone suggests selective inferior vestibular neuritis (Fig. 4C,F,I).

Semicircular Canal Occlusion

Benign paroxysmal positional vertigo (BPV) is caused by lithiasis in the SCCs whereby misplaced otoconia inappropriately stimulate receptor hair cells in response to changes in head position. It has been shown to affect any combination of the three SCCs [49]. In cases of intractable posterior SCC BPV not relieved by particle repositioning manoeuvres [50,51], surgical SCC plugging has been used to occlude the affected SCC to ablate its function. SCC plugging has been most commonly used to occlude the posterior canal [52,53], but also for the lateral canal [54] and anterior canal [55].

Figure 5 shows the head and eye velocity in response to head impulses in two patients who had undergone SCC plugging for right posterior canal benign paroxysmal positional vertigo (Fig. 5A,D,G) and left lateral canal benign paroxysmal positional vertigo (Fig. 5B,E,H). Head impulses approximately in the planes of the SCCs show a VOR deficit with VOR gains of about 0.3–0.4 in the occluded right posterior SCC and occluded left lateral SCC, but normal VOR responses from the remaining SCCs. Similarly, lateral semicircular canal occlusion in animals also demonstrated permanent VOR changes [56].

Superior Canal Dehiscence

Superior (anterior) canal dehiscence is a bony defect in the anterior canal roof leading to hypersensitivity of the vestibular and cochlear receptors to sound and

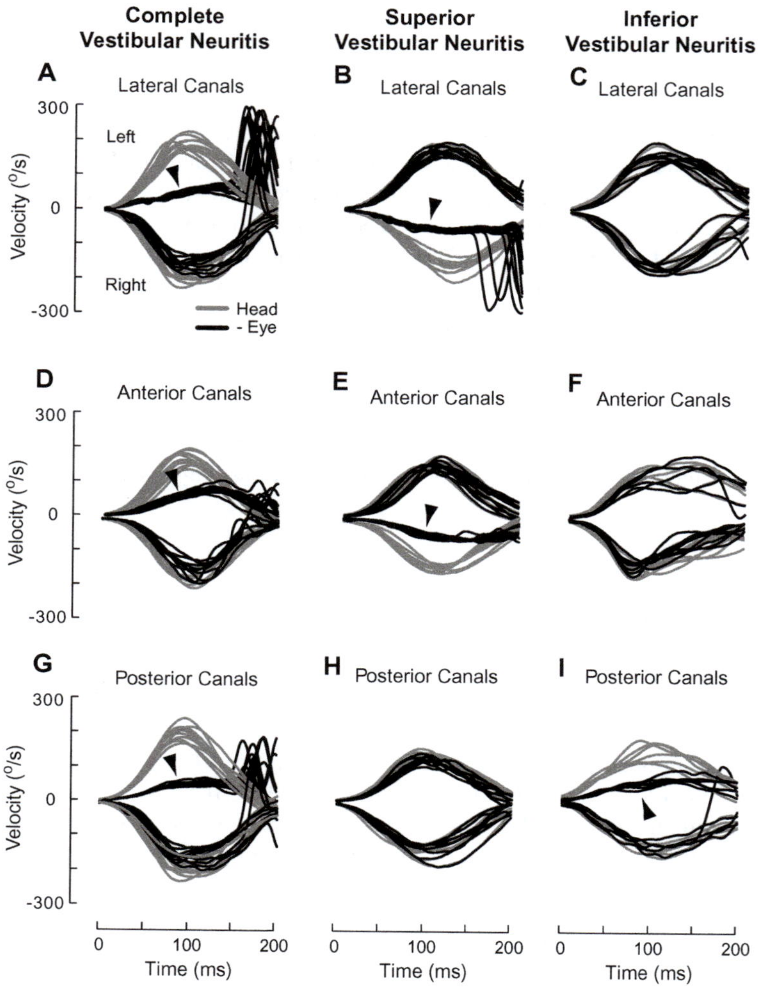

Fig. 4. Examples of yaw, LARP, and RALP head impulses in three patients after vestibular neuritis. **A, D, G** Complete vestibular neuritis involving both the left superior and inferior vestibular nerves results in deficits in the left lateral, superior, and posterior semicircular canals (*arrows*). **B, E, H** Vestibular neuritis of the right superior vestibular nerve leads to right lateral and superior canal deficits (**B, E**; *arrows*). **C, F, I** Vestibular neuritis of the left inferior vestibular nerve only involves the left posterior canal (**I**; *arrow*)

raised middle ear or intracranial pressure. Clinical manifestations comprise vertigo, oscillopsia, nystagmus induced by loud sounds, hearing loss, hyperacusis, and autophony [57–63]. The head impulse test of anterior canal function is often normal, but hypofunction may be present (Fig. 5F), especially if the dehiscence length is 5 mm or more [64,65]. The outcomes of the surgical anterior canal plugging or canal reroofing [59,62,66,67] to provide relief of the signs and

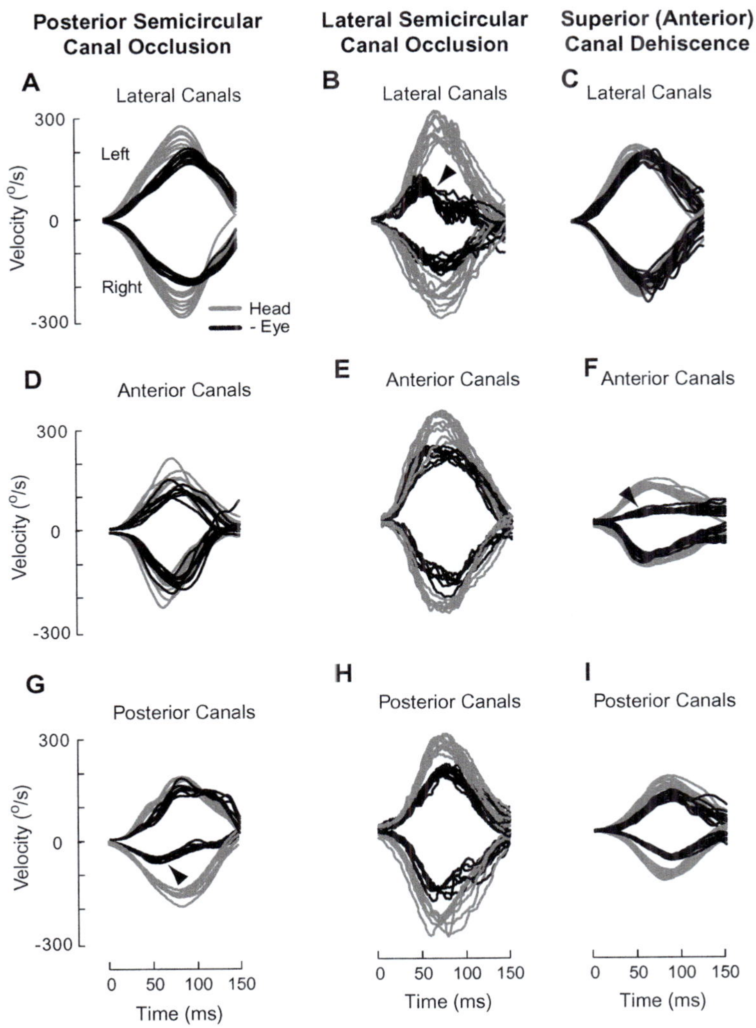

Fig. 5. Examples of three-dimensional head impulses of patients with right posterior SCC occlusion (**A, D, G**), left lateral semicircular canal occlusion (**B, E, H**), and left superior canal dehiscence (unoperated) (**C, F, I**). In head impulses directed toward the inactivated right posterior canal (**G**), the inactivated left lateral canal (**B**), or the dehiscent left superior canal (**F**), the VOR is deficient (*arrows*). However, head impulses directed toward any of the five intact semicircular canals elicited close to normal VOR responses in all patients

symptoms of superior canal dehiscence can be measured with the head impulse test. Both surgical procedures reduce the function of the operated anterior canal but usually preserve the function of the other ipsilateral semicircular canals [68].

The head impulse test can also be used to assess unintended destruction to the rest of the SCCs in any surgical interference of the labyrinth [62] including cochlear implantation, which has been shown to carry a low risk of destruction of SCC function [69].

Meniere's Disease

Meniere's disease is characterized by fluctuating sensorineural hearing loss, aural fullness, tinnitus, episodic vertigo, and nystagmus [70]. In patients with active Meniere's disease, monitoring of the SCC function using the head impulse test does not appear to provide a useful index for the severity of the disease, as individual SCC function can be relatively well preserved and comparable to normal values [10]. However, the head impulse test is useful for monitoring the efficacy of treatment after intratympanic gentamicin [10] or selective vestibular neurectomy with preservation of hearing [26,71].

Monitoring of the VOR gains derived from head impulse tests provides a qualitative and quantitative index of individual SCC functional ablation following intratympanic gentamicin treatment [10,72]. After a single injection of intratympanic gentamicin, the VOR gains of the treated SCCs in response to the head impulse tests are lowered to about 0.4, suggesting that partial ablation of SCC function is sufficient to control vertigo in the majority of Meniere's patients [10].

Some Meniere's disease patients continued to report vertiginous Meniere attacks of lesser severity after selective vestibular neurectomy with sparing of the cochlear nerve [26,73]. Because of anatomic variation of the vestibular nerve topography from the nerve's origin in the internal auditory canal fundus to its entry point at the brainstem [74], some inferior vestibular nerve fibers may cross over to the cochlear nerve and may be spared during selective vestibular neurectomy [73].

The head impulse test is a useful index for quantification of any residual posterior canal function (Fig. 6F), indicating possible sparing of inferior vestibular nerve fibers during selective vestibular neurectomy [26]. The presence of this residual posterior canal function also corroborates with magnetic resonance imaging (MRI) findings of residual bulk and signal suggestive of the inferior vestibular nerve fibers during imaging of the vestibulo-cochlear and facial nerves in the internal auditory canal [71].

Systemic Gentamicin Vestibulotoxicity

Parenteral gentamicin is a cheap and effective antibiotic for life-threatening gram-negative infections with the rare, but potentially devastating, risk of vestibulotoxicity [75,76]. The head impulse test can either clinically monitor the development of vestibular hypofunction at the bedside by visually detecting the refixation saccade [4,38,40,72] or be used with dual-search coils to provide a quantitative assessment of any bilateral vestibular hypofunction [13].

Fig. 6. Three-dimensional head impulse tests of two patients with Meniere's disease after selective vestibular neurectomy with preservation of hearing. The patient after complete selective vestibular neurectomy (**A, C, E**) is asymptomatic, while the patient after incomplete selective neurectomy (**B, D, F**) still suffers from vertiginous attacks. Semicircular canal function is normal on the intact left side in both patients. On the operated right side of the asymptomatic Meniere's patient, the VOR gain is abolished in all canals (**A, C, E**). In contrast, on the operated right side of the still symptomatic Meniere's patient, posterior canal function is partially spared (**F**; *arrow*)

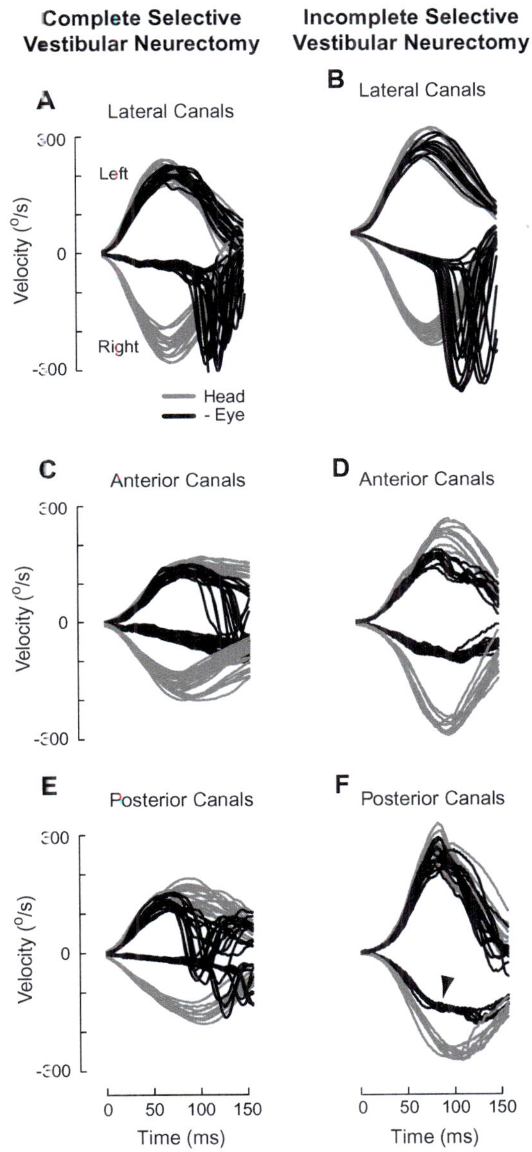

Central Vestibular Lesions

One of the differential diagnoses of acute spontaneous vertigo with a negative head impulse test is acute cerebellar infarction [39] resulting from occlusion of the posterior inferior cerebellar artery. In contrast to a peripheral vestibular lesion, the spontaneous nystagmus may be bilateral, gaze evoked, and change direction, and not suppressed by visual fixation. MR imaging is necessary for confirmation of the diagnosis.

The vestibulocerebellum is thought to play an important role in the calibration of the VOR. This concept is supported by the finding that patients with cerebellar disease showed impaired modulation of both gain and rotation axis of the high-acceleration VOR [77,78].

Acknowledgments Supported by the National Health and Medical Research Council and by the Garnett Passe and Rodney Williams Memorial Foundation.

References

1. Lysakowski A, Goldberg JM (2004) Morphophysiology of the vestibular periphery. In: Highstein SM, Fay RR, Popper AN (eds) The vestibular system. Springer, New York, pp 57–152
2. Ewald EJ (1892) Physiologische Untersuchungen über das Endorgan des Nervus Octavus. Bergmann, Wiesbaden
3. Halmagyi GM, Curthoys IS, Cremer PD, et al (1990a) Head impulses after unilateral vestibular deafferentation validate Ewald's second law. J Vestib Res 1:187–197
4. Halmagyi GM, Curthoys IS (1988) A clinical sign of canal paresis. Arch Neurol 45:737–739
5. Halmagyi GM, Curthoys IS, Cremer PD, et al (1990b) The human horizontal vestibulo-ocular reflex in response to high-acceleration stimulation before and after unilateral vestibular neurectomy. Exp Brain Res 81:479–490
6. Aw ST, Haslwanter T, Halmagyi GM, et al (1996a) Three-dimensional vector analysis of the human vestibuloocular reflex in response to high-acceleration head rotations. I. Responses in normal subjects. J Neurophysiol 76:4009–4020
7. Aw ST, Halmagyi GM, Haslwanter T, et al (1996b) Three-dimensional vector analysis of the human vestibuloocular reflex in response to high-acceleration head rotations. II. Responses in subjects with unilateral vestibular loss and selective semicircular canal occlusion. J Neurophysiol 76:4021–4030
8. Cremer PD, Halmagyi GM, Aw ST, et al (1998) Semicircular canal plane head impulses detect absent function of individual semicircular canals. Brain 121:699–716
9. Schmid-Priscoveanu A, Straumann D, Bohmer A, et al (1999) Vestibulo-ocular responses during static head roll and three dimensional head impulses after vestibular neuritis. Acta Otolaryngol 119:750–757
10. Carey JP, Minor LB, Peng GC, et al (2002) Changes in the three-dimensional angular vestibulo-ocular reflex following intratympanic gentamicin for Meniere's disease. J Assoc Res Otolaryngol 3:430–443
11. Della Santina CC, Cremer PD, Carey JP, et al (2002) Comparison of head thrust test with head autorotation test reveals that the vestibulo-ocular reflex is enhanced during voluntary head movements. Arch Otolaryngol Head Neck Surg 128:1044–1054
12. Black RA, Halmagyi GM, Thurtell MJ, et al (2005) The active head-impulse test in unilateral peripheral vestibulopathy. Arch Neurol 62:290–293
13. Tabak S, Collewijn H, Boumans LJ, et al (1997) Gain and delay of human vestibulo-ocular reflexes to oscillation and steps of the head by a reactive torque helmet. II. Vestibular-deficient subjects. Acta Otolaryngol 117:796–809
14. Collewijn H, Smeets JBJ (2000) Early components of the human vestibulo-ocular response to head rotation: latency and gain. J Neurophysiol 84:376–389

15. Hirvonen M, Aalto H, Migliaccio AA, et al (2007) Motorized head impulse rotator for horizontal vestibulo-ocular reflex: normal responses. Arch Otolaryngol Head Neck Surg 133:157–161
16. Crane BT, Demer JL (1998) Human horizontal vestibulo-ocular reflex initiation: effects of acceleration, target distance, and unilateral deafferentation. J Neurophysiol 80:1151–1166
17. Tian J, Crane BT, Demer JL (2000) Vestibular catch-up saccades in labyrinthine deficiency. Exp Brain Res 131:448–457
18. Tian JR, Ishiyama A, Demer JL (2007) Temporal dynamics of semicircular canal and otolith function following acute unilateral vestibular deafferentation in humans. Exp Brain Res 178:529–541
19. Aw ST, Fetter GM, Halmagyi GM (2001) Individual semicircular canal function in superior and inferior vestibular neuritis. Neurology 57:768–774
20. Hixson WC, Niven JI, Correia MJ (1966) Kinematics nomenclature for physiological accelerations: with special reference to vestibular applications. Monograph 14. Naval Aerospace Medical Research Institute, Pensacola, FL
21. Robinson DA (1963) A method of measuring eye movement using a scleral search coil in a magnetic field. IEEE Trans Biomed Eng 10:137–145
22. Remmel RS (1984) An inexpensive eye movement monitor using the scleral search coil technique. IEEE Trans Biomed Eng 31:388–390
23. Collewijn H, Van der Steen J, Ferman L, et al (1985) Human ocular counterroll: assessment of static and dynamic properties from electromagnetic scleral coil recordings. Exp Brain Res 59:185–196
24. Aw ST, Halmagyi GM, Curthoys IS, et al (1994) Unilateral vestibular deafferentation causes permanent impairment of the human vestibulo-ocular reflex in the pitch plane. Exp Brain Res 102:121–130
25. Aw ST, Halmagyi GM, Pohl DV, et al (1995) Compensation of the human vertical vestibulo-ocular reflex following occlusion of one vertical semicircular canal is incomplete. Exp Brain Res 103:471–475
26. Lehnen N, Aw ST, Todd MJ, et al (2004) Head impulse test reveals residual semicircular canal function after vestibular neurectomy. Neurology 62:2294–2296
27. Bergamin O, Zee DS, Roberts DC, et al (2001) Three-dimensional Hess screen test with binocular dual search coils in a three-field magnetic system. Invest Ophthalmol Vis Sci 42:660–667
28. Haustein W (1989) Considerations on Listing's law and the primary position by means of a matrix description of eye position control. Biol Cybern 60:411–420
29. Haslwanter T (1995) Mathematics of 3-dimensional eye rotations. Vision Res 35:1727–1739
30. Hess BJ, Van Opstal AJ, Straumann D, et al (1992) Calibration of three-dimensional eye position using search coil signals in the rhesus monkey. Vision Res 32:1647–1654
31. Weber KP, Aw ST, Todd MJ, et al (2008) Head impulse test in unilateral vestibular loss: vestibulo-ocular reflex and catch-up saccades. Neurology 70:454–463
32. Bronstein AM, Hood JD (1986) The cervico-ocular reflex in normal subjects and patients with absent vestibular function. Brain Res 373:399–408
33. Kimmig H, Biscaldi M, Mutter J, et al (2002) The initiation of smooth pursuit eye movements and saccades in normal subjects and in "express-saccade makers." Exp Brain Res 144:373–384
34. Minor LB, Lasker DM, Backous DD, et al (1999) Horizontal vestibuloocular reflex evoked by high-acceleration rotations in the squirrel monkey. I. Normal responses. J Neurophysiol 82:1254–1270
35. Migliaccio AA, Schubert MC, Jiradejvong P, et al (2004) The three-dimensional vestibulo-ocular reflex evoked by high-acceleration rotations in the squirrel monkey. Exp Brain Res 159:433–446
36. Blanks RHI, Curthoys IS, Markham CH (1975) Planar relationships of the semicircular canals in man. Acta Otolaryngol 80:185–196

37. Aw ST, Haslwanter T, Fetter M, et al (1998) Contribution of the vertical semicircular canals to the caloric nystagmus. Acta Otolaryngol 118:618–627
38. Benyon GJ, Jani P, Baguley DM (1998) A clinical evaluation of head impulse testing. Clin Otolaryngol 23:117–122
39. Halmagyi GM (2005) Diagnosis and management of vertigo. Clin Med 5:159–165
40. Jorns-Häderli M, Straumann D, Palla A (2007) Accuracy of the bedside head-impulse test in detecting vestibular hypofunction. J Neurol Neurosurg Psychiatry 78:1113–1118
41. Peng GCY, Zee DS, Minor LB (2004) Phase-plane analysis of gaze stabilization to high acceleration head thrusts: a continuum across normal subjects and patients with loss of vestibular function. J Neurophysiol 91:1763–1781
42. Gilchrist DP, Curthoys IS, Cartwright AD, et al (1998) High acceleration impulsive rotations reveal severe long-term deficits of the horizontal vestibulo-ocular reflex in the guinea pig. Exp Brain Res 123:242–254
43. Curthoys IS, Topple AN, Halmagyi GM (1995) Unilateral vestibular deafferentation (UVD) causes permanent asymmetry in the gain of the yaw VOR to high acceleration head impulses in guinea pigs. Acta Otolaryngol Suppl 520:59–61
44. Sadeghi SG, Minor LB, Cullen KE (2006) Dynamics of the horizontal vestibuloocular reflex after unilateral labyrinthectomy: response to high frequency, high acceleration, and high velocity rotations. Exp Brain Res 175:471–484
45. Fetter M, Dichgans J (1996) Vestibular neuritis spares the inferior division of the vestibular nerve. Brain 119:755–763
46. Strupp M, Brandt T (1999) Vestibular neuritis. In: Buttner U (ed) Vestibular dysfunction and its therapy. Adv Otorhinolaryngol 55:111–136
47. Schmid-Priscoveanu A, Bohmer A, Obzina H, et al (2001) Caloric and search-coil head-impulse testing in patients after vestibular neuritis. J Assoc Res Otolaryngol 2:72–78
48. Palla A, Straumann D (2004) Recovery of the high-acceleration vestibulo-ocular reflex after vestibular neuritis. J Assoc Res Otolaryngol 5:427–435
49. Aw ST, Todd MJ, Aw GE, et al (2005) Benign positional nystagmus: a study of its three-dimensional spatio-temporal characteristics. Neurology 64:1897–1905
50. Epley JM (2001) Human experience with canalith repositioning maneuvers. Ann N Y Acad Sci 942:179–191
51. Semont A, Freyss G, Vitte E (1988) Curing the BPPV with a liberatory maneuver. Adv Otorhinolaryngol 42:290–293
52. Parnes LS, McClure JA (1990) Posterior semicircular canal occlusion for intractable benign paroxysmal positional vertigo. Ann Otol Rhinol Laryngol 99:330–334
53. Parnes LS, McClure JA (1992) Free-floating endolymph particles: a new operative finding during posterior semicircular canal occlusion. Laryngoscope 102:988–992
54. Agrawal SK, Parnes LS (2001) Human experience with canal plugging. Ann N Y Acad Sci 942:300–305
55. Brantberg K, Bergenius J (2002) Treatment of anterior benign paroxysmal positional vertigo by canal plugging: a case report. Acta Otolaryngol 122:28–30
56. Gilchrist DP, Curthoys IS, Burgess AM, et al (2000) Semicircular canal occlusion causes permanent VOR changes. Neuroreport 11:2527–2531
57. Minor LB, Solomon D, Zinreich JS, et al (1998) Sound- and/or pressure-induced vertigo due to bone dehiscence of the superior semicircular canal. Arch Otolaryngol Head Neck Surg 124:249–258
58. Cremer PD, Minor LB, Carey JP, et al (2000) Eye movements in patients with superior semicircular canal dehiscence align with the abnormal canal. Neurology 55:1833–1841
59. Brantberg K, Bergenius J, Mendel L, et al (2001) Symptoms, findings and treatment in patients with dehiscence of the superior semicircular canal. Acta Otolaryngol 121:68–75
60. Halmagyi GM, Aw ST, McGarvie LA, et al (2003) Superior semicircular canal dehiscence simulating otosclerosis. J Laryngol Otol 117:553–557
61. Mikulec AA, McKenna MJ, Ramsey MJ, et al (2004) Superior semicircular canal dehiscence presenting as conductive hearing loss without vertigo. Otol Neurotol 25:121–129

62. Minor LB (2005) Clinical manifestations of superior semicircular canal dehiscence. Laryngoscope 115:1717–1727
63. Aw ST, Todd MJ, Aw GE, et al (2006a) Click-evoked vestibulo-ocular reflex: stimulus-response properties in superior canal dehiscence. Neurology 66:1079–1087
64. Minor LB, Cremer PD, Carey JP, et al (2001) Symptoms and signs in superior canal dehiscence syndrome. Ann N Y Acad Sci 942:259–273
65. Deutschländer A, Strupp M, Jahn K, et al (2004) Vertical oscillopsia in bilateral superior canal dehiscence syndrome. Neurology 62:784–787
66. Minor LB (2000) Superior canal dehiscence syndrome. Am J Otol 21:9–19
67. Mikulec AA, Poe DS, McKenna MJ (2005) Operative management of superior semicircular canal dehiscence. Laryngoscope 115:501–507
68. Carey JP, Migliaccio AA, Minor LB (2007) Semicircular canal function before and after surgery for superior canal dehiscence. Otol Neurotol 28:356–364
69. Migliaccio AA, Della Santina CC, Carey JP, et al (2005) The vestibulo-ocular reflex response to head impulses rarely decreases after cochlear implantation. Otol Neurotol 26:655–660
70. Minor LB, Schessel DA, Carey JP (2004) Meniere's disease. Curr Opin Neurol 17:9–16
71. Aw ST, Magnussen JS, Todd MJ, et al (2006b) MRI of the vestibular nerve after selective vestibular neurectomy. Acta Otolaryngol 126:1053–1056
72. Casani A, Nuti D, Franceschini SS, et al (2005) Transtympanic gentamicin and fibrin tissue adhesive for treatment of unilateral Meniere's disease: effects on vestibular function. Otolaryngol Head Neck Surg 133:929–935
73. Silverstein H, Jackson LE (2002) Vestibular nerve section. Otolaryngol Clin N Am 35: 655–673
74. Terasaka S, Sawamura Y, Fukushima T (2000) Topography of the vestibulocochlear nerve. Neurosurgery 47:162–168
75. Halmagyi GM, Fattore CM, Curthoys IS, et al (1994) Gentamicin vestibulotoxicity. Otolaryngol Head Neck Surg 111:571–574
76. Black FO, Pesznecker S, Stallings V (2004) Permanent gentamicin vestibulotoxicity. Otol Neurotol 25:559–569
77. Crane BT, Tian JR, Demer JL (2000) Initial vestibulo-ocular reflex during transient angular and linear acceleration in human cerebellar dysfunction. Exp Brain Res 130:486–496
78. Walker MF, Zee DS (2005) Cerebellar disease alters the axis of the high-acceleration vestibuloocular reflex. J Neurophysiol 94:3417–3429

Part V
Neurological Cases

Similarities and Differences Between Auditory Neuropathy and Acoustic Neuroma

Tatsuya Yamasoba

Summary

We evaluated auditory function in 50 patients with unilateral acoustic neuroma. By comparing pure tone audiometric thresholds and distortion product otoacoustic emissions, we classified their hearing impairment into three categories: neural hearing loss (group I, $n = 7$), mixture of neural and cochlear hearing loss (group II, $n = 5$), and cochlear hearing loss (group III, $n = 38$). In auditory brainstem response (ABR) examinations, only wave I was present in group I; group II exhibited wave I alone or no waves; and in group III, all waves were present in patients with mild deafness, delayed waves III and V or wave V alone in those with moderate deafness, and no responses in those with profound deafness. Tone decay was observed only in groups I and II, whereas recruitment phenomena were present only in group III. Speech discrimination was poor and out of proportion to the pure tone audiometric configuration in groups I and II, whereas it corresponded well with the degree of hearing loss in group III. These findings indicate that ABR wave I alone, tone decay, and poor speech discrimination are characteristic to neural hearing loss associated with acoustic neuroma. The differences and similarities between auditory neuropathy and acoustic neuroma are discussed.

Key words Acoustic neuroma, Otoacoustic emission, Tone decay, Speech perception, Auditory brainstem response

Introduction

Hearing loss is the most frequent symptom in acoustic neuroma. However, the exact mechanism of hearing loss associated with acoustic neuroma. is not certain.

Department of Otolaryngology, and Head and Neck Surgery, The University of Tokyo, 7-3-1 Hongo, Bunkyo-ku, Tokyo 113-8655, Japan

doi: 10.1007/978-4-431-09433-3_12,

Schuknecht [1] listed three major causes: (1) destruction of cochlear and vestibular nerve fibers, (2) destruction of sense organs as a result of the ischemia caused by the tumor, and (3) biochemical disturbances in the inner ear fluids. Direct invasion of the cochlea by tumor, although rare, can also cause hearing loss. Because of this variety of causes, hearing loss caused by acoustic neuroma may involve the cochlea, the retrocochlear auditory pathway, or both, producing a complex and varied picture of auditory symptoms and signs.

Evoked otoacoustic emissions (OAEs) arise from a stimulus-induced release of acoustic energy from the cochlea into the external ear canal. The active cochlear processing is considered to originate in the miniscule movements of the outer hair cells. Two different types of OAEs, transiently (click) evoked OAEs (TEOAEs) and distortion product OAEs (DPOAEs), have been widely used to detect cochlear hearing loss in humans because these emissions can be clearly recorded in nearly all subjects with normal cochlear and middle ear function [2–4]. The relationship between the amplitude of TEOAE frequency spectrum and the extent of hearing loss is complex, because the amplitude of TEOAEs in a given spectral band is dependent on not only hearing threshold within the band but that outside the band as well [5]. In contrast, because of the pure tone features of their evoking stimuli, DPOAEs have the ability to be elicited at any test frequency, especially frequencies between 0.8 and 8 kHz. It has been shown that DPOAEs elicited by two primary tones, f1 and f2, correlate well with hearing thresholds at their geometric mean frequency [6,7]. In addition, DPOAEs are more robust than TEOAEs in the presence of mild to moderate cochlear hearing loss [4,6,8]. TEOAEs cannot be recorded in patients with hearing thresholds greater than 40 dB HL at the best hearing frequency [2,5], whereas DPOAEs can usually be measured in ears exhibiting cochlear hearing loss up to 65 dB HL [4,6]. In our previous study using primary tones f1 and f2 at 70 dB SPL, DPOAE could be detected in ears with hearing threshold less than 50 dB HL at 1 kHz and 2 kHz and 65 dB HL or less at 4 kHz [6]. Because of these features, DPOAEs are considered more suitable than TEOAEs to separate and identify cochlear deafness from neural deafness induced by acoustic neuroma [9].

To differentiate cochlear deafness from neural deafness, it is necessary to compare DPOAE amplitude features to the related hearing thresholds. For example, hearing loss is considered to involve the cochlea when DPOAEs are undetected or reduced as expected from the extent of hearing loss at the frequency related to the DPOAEs. When ears with hearing loss exhibit DPOAEs with normal range, the hearing loss is considered to result from neural damage. When DPOAE levels are reduced but better than expected from the extent of hearing losses or when DPOAE levels are within normal range at some frequencies but impaired at other frequencies, it is considered that both neural and cochlear damage exist. Using this criterion, in the current study, we classified hearing in ears with acoustic neuroma into three categories: neural, mixed (i.e., mixture of neural and cochlear damage), and cochlear hearing loss. We studied auditory findings in acoustic neuroma patients in each category and compared them to those in patients with auditory neuropathy.

Patients and Methods

Patients

Of patients who visited our deafness clinic in Department of Otolaryngology and Head and Neck Surgery, University of Tokyo, we included 50 patients who fulfilled the following criteria: (1) the presence of unilateral acoustic neuroma was surgically confirmed, (2) there was no evidence of other neurological disease or brain lesions, (3) there was no history of middle or inner ear disease in either ear, and (4) the amplitude of DPOAE evoked in the contralateral ear was within normal range. The patients ranged from 13 to 68 years in age (average, 45 years old). Informed consent was obtained from the participants after the nature of the procedures had been fully explained.

Audiological Examinations

Audiological examinations included pure tone audiometry, speech discrimination, Bekesy's audiometry, Fowler's alternate binaural loudness balance testing, short intermittent sensitivity index test (SISI), acoustic reflex testing, DPOAEs, and auditory brainstem response (ABR) measurement. All testing was performed inside an electrically shielded sound-attenuating room.

DPOAEs were recorded and analyzed in bilateral ears using an ILO 92 (ver. 1.31) Otodynamic Analyzer. Primary tones f1 and f2 were presented at 70 dB SPL. The f2/f1 ratio was kept at approximately 1.22 (range, 1.21–1.23), and the frequency was changed in 1/4 octave steps from 708 Hz to 6299 Hz. The levels of the DPOAEs at 2f1-f2 were recorded. The distortion product (DP)-gram illustrated the relationship between the amplitudes of the 2f1-f2 DPOAEs and the geometric mean of f1 and f2 frequency. The measurement at 2f1-f2 was considered significantly different from background noise if it exceeded the average noise level by at least two standard deviations. Normal range (average ± 1 SD) for DPOAE amplitudes was obtained in 40 normal subjects (80 ears). To compare DPOAE features in ears with acoustic neuroma to those in ears with cochlear hearing loss, we also measured DPOAEs in 150 ears exhibiting cochlear hearing loss such as noise-induced deafness (cochlear damage controls).

ABR was recorded with silver disk electrodes from the forehead, referenced to the test ear mastoid, and grounded to the opposite ear mastoid. The acoustic stimuli were alternating polarity clicks (0.1-ms rectangular pulse) with the intensity of 90 dB HL. The contralateral ear was masked with white noise of 70 dB HL. One thousand sweeps were averaged twice with bandpass filters at 150 and 3000 Hz, 6 dB/octave. Latencies of wave I, III, and V and the interpeak latencies I–III, III–V, and I–V were measured and compared with institutional normative data.

Criteria to Determine the Site Responsible for Hearing Loss

To differentiate cochlear hearing loss from neural hearing loss, we compared DPOAE amplitude features to hearing thresholds at the related frequency (i.e., the geometric mean of two primary tones f1 and f2). In this manner, ears with behaviorally measured hearing losses (i.e., hearing thresholds greater than 20 dB HL) and DPOAE amplitudes that were reduced or undetected as expected from impaired hearing were assigned to a cochlear loss group. Ears with behaviorally hearing losses and DPOAE amplitudes within normal range were assigned to a neural loss group. Ears in which DPOAE amplitudes were reduced but better than expected from the extent of hearing losses (better than those found in cochlear damage controls) or those in which DPOAE levels were within normal range at some frequencies but reduced as expected from impaired hearing at other frequencies were assigned to a mixed loss group (a group with mixture of neural and cochlear hearing loss).

Results

By comparing hearing thresholds and DPOAE amplitude features, 7 tumor ears (14%) were assigned to a neural hearing loss group, 5 (10%) to a mixed hearing loss group, and 38 (76%) to a cochlear loss group. In other words, of 50 tumor ears with hearing loss, the retrocochlear neural elements were involved in 12 (24%), whereas the cochlea was involved in 43 (86%).

As to the relationship between DPOAE amplitudes and hearing thresholds at their related frequencies, ears in the neural loss groups exhibited DPOAEs with amplitudes within normal range. In the mixed loss group, DPOAE amplitudes were reduced similarly to cochlear damage controls in two ears only at 1 kHz and in one ear only at 2 and 4 kHz, whereas the remaining ears exhibited DPOAE amplitudes that were reduced but significantly better than expected from the extent of hearing loss (i.e., better than cochlear damage controls). In the cochlear hearing loss group, DPOAEs were detected at least at one frequency in ten ears with milder hearing loss (9 ears at 1 kHz, 5 ears at 2 kHz, and 8 ears at 4 kHz). In these ears, the DPOAE amplitude reduction correlated well with the extent of hearing loss, as were cochlear damage controls. DPOAEs were not detected (under noise floor) in the remaining ears, in which hearing impairment was moderate to profound.

Recruitment phenomenon that was evaluated with SISI, acoustic reflex testing, and Bekesy's audiometry was present in 34 ears in the cochlear loss group. None in the other groups showed recruitment phenomenon. Tone decay was evident in 5 ears in the neural loss group and 4 ears in the mixed loss group; the presence of tone decay could not be evaluated in the remaining ears in these groups because of totally deafness at the frequencies examined. None in the cochlear hearing loss groups exhibited tone decay.

Table 1. Auditory brainstem response (ABR) findings in 50 patients with unilateral acoustic neuroma

	No waves	Wave I alone	Wave V (+III)	All waves
Neural damage		7		
Neural and cochlear damage	3	2		
Cochlear damage	8		13	17

In the cochlear hearing loss group, speech discrimination score (SDS) correlated well with the extent of hearing loss; SDS grew worse as hearing thresholds increased. In contrast, the neural and mixed loss groups showed very poor speech discrimination, mostly less than 20%, regardless of their hearing thresholds. SDS was significantly worse in these groups compared to the cochlear loss group.

No ears showed normal ABR waveforms with normal peak and interpeak latencies, and thus ABR findings were classified into four categories: (1) absence of all waves; (2) wave I alone with the later waves absent; (3) delayed wave V or waves III and V with wave I absent; and (4) all waves present with prolonged interpeak latencies. Table 1 summarizes ABR findings in the three groups. All ears in the neural loss group exhibited the presence of wave I alone. In the mixed hearing loss group, only wave I was present in two ears and no waveforms were elicited in three ears. In the cochlear hearing loss group, ABR findings correlated well with the extent of hearing loss. Ears with milder hearing loss showed all waves with prolonged interpeak latencies between waves I and III and I and V. As hearing thresholds increased, wave I became undetectable and delayed wave V with or without waves III was recorded. When hearing loss became profound, no clear waves were observed.

Discussion

Audiological Characteristics in Cochlear and Neural Hearing Loss Associated with Acoustic Neuroma

By comparing hearing thresholds and DPOAE amplitude features, the current study demonstrated that hearing loss induced by acoustic neuroma more frequently involved the cochlea than the retrocochlear neural elements. Of 50 acoustic neuroma patients, the retrocochlear neural elements were involved in 12 patients (24%) and the cochlea in 43 patients (86%).

Bonfils and Uziel [10] reported that TEOAEs were recorded in 9 of 28 patients with surgically proven acoustic neuroma and that the incidence of TEOAEs highly correlated with hearing thresholds. In this study, two subjects (7%) showed an unexpected presence of TEOAEs with regard to their elevated hearing thresholds, which is compatible with neural damage. Similarly, Pröschel et al. [11] found that in 31 (91%) of the 34 acoustic neuroma patients, the spectrum of the TEOAEs corresponded well with the pure tone audiometric configuration; however, 3 (9%) showed good emissions in spite of a demonstrable hearing loss, suggestive of neural hearing loss. Prasher et al. [12] reported that TEOAE was recorded in 7 of 26 acoustic neuroma ears in which hearing was better than 40 dB HL in the region of 0.5 to 2 kHz. No TEOAEs were recorded in the remaining ears, in which hearing at 1 and 2 kHz was greater than 30 and 40 dB HL, respectively. Using DPOAEs and TEOAEs, Telischi et al. [9] found that hearing loss involved the cochlea in 71% and neural elements in 41% of 44 patients with surgically verified acoustic neuroma. Later, by comparing preoperative pure tone audiometric configurations and DPOAEs in 97 patients with surgically confirmed acoustic neuroma, Telischi [13] assigned 55 (57%) of the tumor ears to the cochlear damage group, 40 (41%) to the noncochlear damage group, and 2 (2%) to an indeterminate group. Although the proportion of cochlear versus neural involvement in acoustic neuroma somewhat differed among reports, mainly because the different modality of testing used, the cochlea appears to be more frequently involved.

The current study also demonstrated that abnormal DPOAEs and impaired speech perception that correspond well to the extent of hearing loss, abnormal ABR beginning with wave I, and the presence of recruitment phenomenon are characteristic to cochlear hearing loss associated with acoustic neuroma. In contrast, normal DPOAEs, the presence of ABR wave I alone, the presence of tone decay, and very poor speech discrimination are indicative of neural hearing loss. The findings observed in the neural hearing loss group are compatible to the pathology existing in the proximal portion of the cochlear nerve, brainstem, or both.

Audiological Characteristics in Auditory Neuropathy

Auditory neuropathy [14] or auditory nerve disease [15] was initially described as impairment of auditory neural function, with preserved cochlear hair cell function, independently by two groups. Since then, the term auditory neuropathy has been used for a variety of individuals (mostly children) who fulfill the following criteria: (1) significant difficulty in speech comprehension, especially in noise, that is out of proportion to the behavioral pure tone audiometric configuration; (2) evidence of normal or nearly normal outer hair cell function (recordable OAE and/or cochlear microphonics); and (3) physiological evidence of impaired auditory neural function (absent or atypical ABRs beginning with wave I) [13–17].

Auditory neuropathy has appeared to consist of a number of varieties, with different etiologies and sites affected. Multiple possible etiologies for auditory neuropathy have been proposed, including genetic, toxic, and metabolic factors, anoxia, hyperbilirubinemia, and mitochondrial disorders [17]. The hearing loss in auditory neuropathy ranges from mild to profound, and most losses are bilateral and symmetrical in configuration [16]. Audiometric configurations are usually flat; however, a smaller but noticeable percentage displays a rising audiometric configuration (i.e., poorer threshold in the low-frequency regions than the high). Speech perception is significantly impaired, especially in noise, and tone decay is evident.

The particulars of the disrupted auditory nerve activity in auditory neuropathy are still unclear, but it is known that it accompanies disorders of the auditory nerve (postsynaptic) and disorders of inner hair cells and their synapses with cochlear nerve terminal (presynaptic). McMahon et al. [18] reported two dominant patterns of frequency-specific round window electrocochleogram (ECochG) waveforms produced by a high-frequency alternating tone burst in patients with profound deafness associated with auditory neuropathy: (1) gross waveform showing a prolonged summating potential (SP) latency followed by a small compound action potential (CAP); and (2) gross waveform showing a normal latency SP waveform followed by a broad negative potential (assumed to reflect the dendritic potential identified in anesthetized guinea pigs). The former suggests a presynaptic disorder and the latter a postsynaptic one. In most subjects showing the first ECochG pattern, electrically evoked ABRs with normal morphology were elicited, whereas all subjects showing the second ECochG pattern, exhibiting electrically evoked ABR waveforms that were absent or having poor wave V morphology. Another recent study using transtympanic ECochG [19] revealed three patterns of cochlear potentials in auditory neuropathy as follows: (1) presence of receptor SP without CAP consistent with presynaptic disorder of inner hair cells; (2) presence of both SP and CAP consistent with postsynaptic disorder of proximal auditory nerve; and (3) presence of prolonged neural potentials without a CAP consistent with postsynaptic disorder of nerve terminals.

Similarities and Differences Between Auditory Neuropathy and Neural Deafness in Acoustic Neuroma

Table 2 summarizes the characteristics of auditory findings in cochlear and neural loss associated with acoustic neuroma and auditory neuropathy. Hearing loss is mostly bilateral and symmetrical in acoustic neuroma, whereas acoustic neuroma involves unilateral ear except when it is associated with neurofibromatosis. Audiograms vary widely in acoustic neuroma, whereas it is predominantly flat, followed by a rising auditory configuration. When auditory neuropathy and neural loss in acoustic neuroma are compared, there are several similarities in their auditory test results; these include the presence of tone decay, normal DPOAEs and cochlear microphonics, and poor speech perception that is out of proportion to the pure tone audiometric configuration. In contrast, the pattern of abnormalities in ABR was markedly different between acoustic neuroma and auditory neuropathy. Neural loss in acoustic neuroma commonly exhibits only wave I, with the following waves absent, whereas in auditory neuropathy, ABR is usually absent and, when present, the abnormalities begin with wave I. This difference in ABR findings may be explained by the difference of the involved sites in acoustic neuroma and auditory neuropathy.

Table 2. Characteristics in auditory findings in acoustic neuroma and auditory neuropathy

	Acoustic neuroma		
	Cochlear hearing loss	Neural hearing loss	Auditory neuropathy
Involvement	Mostly unilateral	Mostly unilateral	Mostly bilateral
Audiometric configuration	No predominant pattern	No predominant pattern	Predominantly flat, followed by low tone loss
Speech perception	Correlating with the degree of hearing loss	Poor	Poor
Tone decay	Absent	Present	Present
Recruitment phenomenon	Present	Absent	Absent
DPOAE	Abnormal	Normal	Normal
ABR	Varying depending on the degree of hearing loss	Wave I alone	Absent or abnormal, beginning with wave I

DPOAE, distortion product otoacoustic emissions; ABR, auditory brainstem response

References

1. Schuknecht HF (1974) Pathology of the ear. Harvard University Press, Cambridge, pp 425–436
2. Probst R, Lonsbury-Martin BL, Martin GK (1991) A review of otoacoustic emissions. J Acoust Soc Am 89:2027–2067
3. Martin GK, Probst R, Lonsbury-Martin BL (1990) Otoacoustic emissions in human ears. Normative findings. Ear Hear 11:106–120
4. Moulin A, Bera JC, Collet L (1994) Distortion product otoacoustic emissions and sensorineural hearing loss. Audiology 33:305–326
5. Collet L, Veuillet E, Chanal JM, et al (1991) Evoked otoacoustic emissions. Correlates between spectrum analysis and audiogram. Audiology 30:164–172
6. Nakamura M, Yamasoba T, Kaga K (1997) Changes in otoacoustic emissions in patients with idiopathic sudden deafness. Audiology 36:121–135
7. Martin GK, Ohlms LA, Franklin DJ, et al (1990) Distortion product emissions in humans. III. Influence of sensorineural hearing loss. Ann Otol Rhinol Laryngol 147:30–42
8. Lonsbury-Martin BL, Whitehead ML, Martin GK (1991) Clinical applications of otoacoustic emissions. J Speech Hear Res 34:964–981
9. Telischi FF, Roth J, Stagner BB, et al (1995) Patterns of evoked otoacoustic emissions associated with acoustic neuromas. Laryngoscope 105:675–682.
10. Bonfils P, Uziel A (1988) Evoked otoacoustic emissions in patients with acoustic neurinomas. Am J Otol 9:412–417
11. Pröschel U, Eysholdt U, Berg M (1994) Transitory evoked otoacoustic emissions in patients with cerebellopontile angle tumors. HNO 42:229–232
12. Prasher DK, Tun T, Brookes GB, et al (1995) Mechanisms of hearing loss in acoustic neuroma. An otoacoustic emission study. Acta Otolaryngol (Stockh) 115:375–381
13. Telischi F (2000) An objective method of analyzing cochlear versus noncochlear patterns of distortion-product otoacoustic emissions in patients with acoustic neuromas. Laryngoscope 110:553–562
14. Starr A, Picton TW, Sininger Y, et al (1996) Auditory neuropathy. Brain 119:741–753

15. Kaga K, Nakamura M, Shinogami M (1996) Auditory nerve disease of both ears revealed by auditory brainstem responses, electrocochleography and otoacoustic emissions. Scand Audiol 25:233–238
16. Rapin I, Gravel J (2003) "Auditory neuropathy": physiologic and pathologic evidence calls for more diagnostic specificity. Int J Pediatr Otorhinolaryngol 67:707–728
17. Raveh E, Buller N, Badrana O, et al (2007) Auditory neuropathy: clinical characteristics and therapeutic approach. Am J Otolaryngol 28:302–308
18. McMahon CM, Patuzzi RB, Gibson WP, et al (2008) Frequency-specific electrocochleography indicates that presynaptic and postsynaptic mechanisms of auditory neuropathy exist. Ear Hear 29:314–325
19. Santarelli R, Starr A, Michalewski HJ, et al (2008) Neural and receptor cochlear potentials obtained by transtympanic electrocochleography in auditory neuropathy. Clin Neurophysiol 119:1028–1041

Diagnosis of Auditory Neuropathy (AN) in Child Neurology

Makiko Kaga[1,2], Masumi Inagaki[1,2], Kaori Kon[1], Akira Uno[1], and Tatsuro Nobutoki[2]

Summary

Discrepancy of normal hearing and auditory brainstem response (ABR) abnormality has been a focus of attention since the early stages of the introduction of ABR to clinical medicine. The concept of auditory neuropathy (AN) seems to be in chaos because AN should be a syndrome with various etiologies and clinical features with mutual discrepancy in neurophysiolcgical findings of ABR and otoacoustic emission (OAE). In this situation, we have found three patients with almost no ABR and normal OAE in our child neurclogy clinic. Among these three patients, the pure type of AN was diagnosed only in one patient, and for the other two patients the diagnoses were "fluctuating hearing loss, episodic headache, and stroke with platelet hyperaggregability" and "alternating hemiplegia of childhood (AHC)." Thus, we would like to recommend that patients who have pure auditory nerve symptoms and are suspected of localized pathology in the auditory nerve should be named as having "auditory nerve disease (AND)" and patients with other complicated physical symptoms should be diagnosed as "auditory neuropathy (AN)" as the special symptom of the underlying diseases.

Key words Auditory neuropathy, Auditory nerve disease, Auditory agnosia, Pure word deafness, Delayed speech

Introduction

Discrepancy of normal hearing and auditory brainstem response (ABR) abnormality has been a focus of attention since the early stage of the introduction of ABR to clinical medicine [1–3]. The first report of auditory neuropathy (AN) by Starr et al. [4] in 1996 included three patients with Charcot–Marie–Tooth disease (CMTD), five patients with some neurological symptoms, and two patients with apparently

[1]Department of Developmental Disorders, National Institute of Mental Health, National Center of Neurology and Psychiatry (NCNP), 4-1-1 Ogawa-Higashi, Kodaira, Tokyo 187-8553, Japan

[2]Division of Child Neurology, National Center Hospital, National Center of Neurology and Psychiatry (NCNP), 4-1-1 Ogawa-Higashi, Kodaira, Tokyo 187-8553, Japan

doi: 10.1007/978-4-431-09433-3_13,

auditory symptoms. It has been suggested that AN is one of the symptoms of systemic disease. On the other hand, Kaga et al. [5] reported the same category of two patients as auditory nerve disease (AND) with only auditory and vestibular symptoms.

Recent clinical diagnostic criteria of AN often seem to be merely a discrepancy of ABR and otoacoustic emission (OAE). However, it is possible for the concept of AN to fall into chaos without formal audiological examinations, especially in the universal neonatal hearing screening setting [6].

In this situation, we have found three patients with almost no ABR and normal OAE in our child neurology clinic. We present the case reports of these patients and discuss the diagnosis of these syndromes.

Case Reports

Case 1: Seven-Year-Old Boy

His Diagnosis is the Pure Type of AN [7].

His chief complaint was delayed speech and suspicion of auditory verbal agnosia. He was born at full term with uneventful pre-, peri-, and postnatal history. He walked unaided at 11 months of age. He uttered some meaningful words at 18 months, but after that his vocabulary remained the same for a long time. He entered nursery school at 3 years of age and entered mainstream elementary school at 6 years of age. He has received speech training since 4 years of age, and his mother had asked for workup of his delayed speech at several rehabilitation centers since he was 3 years old. At 7 years and 3 months of age, he underwent ABR examination for the first time. The parents were informed that the result was quite abnormal despite his normal hearing acuity.

Thus, he was referred to our hospital for further workup of his auditory condition. He could talk, read aloud, and repeat short sentences. However, he could not fully understand what he was asked, what he had read, and what he repeated by himself. He responded to environmental sounds, but he was slow or sometimes unable to respond to pure verbal commands. Physical and neurological examinations were all normal.

Psychological and Neuropsychological Test Findings

Verbal, performance, and Full-IQs of Wechsler Scale for Children III-R were 53, 118, and 81, respectively. Raven colored matrixes test was normal (33/36). Peabody picture vocabulary test showed his verbal age was at 4 years level. Results of the Illinois Test for Psycholinguistic Ability (ITPA) revealed very poor auditory verbal ability and excellent visual nonverbal ability. Profile of Kaufmann Assessment Battery for Children (K-ABC) disclosed a good reading ability with poor understanding. Those findings suggested semantic impairment of language or auditory verbal agnosia [8,9].

Hearing Acuity and Auditory Perception

Pure tone audiogram was completely normal. His speech discrimination ability was less than 50% at 50–60 dB nHL (Fig. 1). Electrocochleogram, tympanogram, and stapedial reflex were normal. He could identify 22 of 24 environmental sounds with visual matching. However, without visual aids, he could identify only 11 of the same 24 environmental sounds. The dichotic listening test (DLT) did not suggest ear preponderance. By sound localization test [10], he could detect sound intensity difference but not time difference.

Neurophysiological Examinations

ABR showed no response at high sound intensity clicks and tone bursts. Apparent wave I induced by 106 dB SPL alternating clicks was the same as induced by

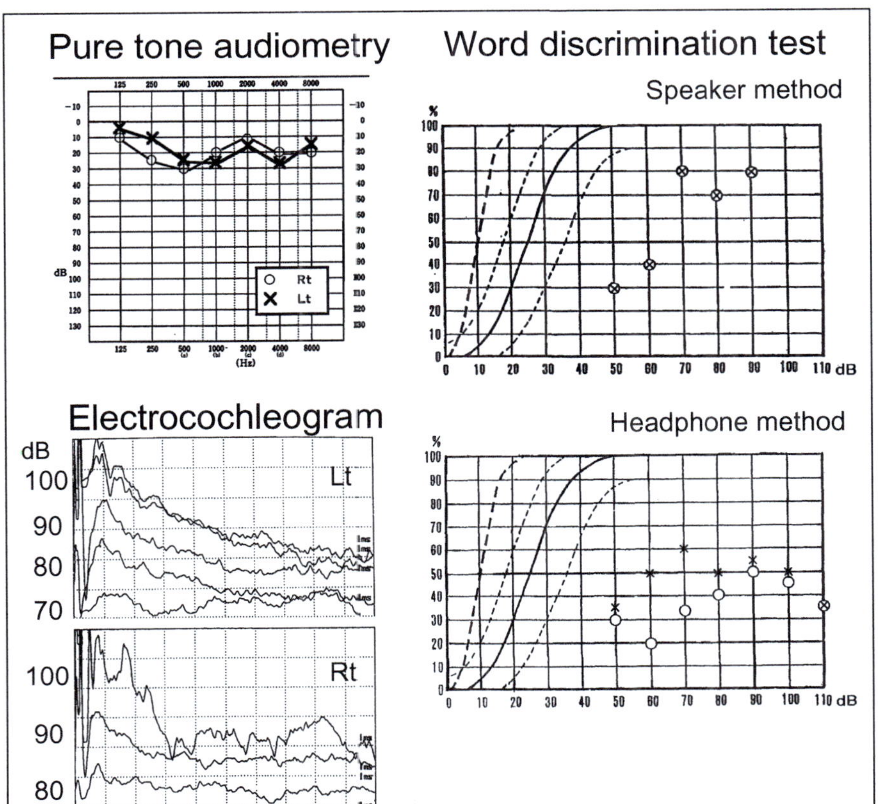

Fig. 1. Pure tone audiogram, word discrimination test, and electrocochleogram of case 1

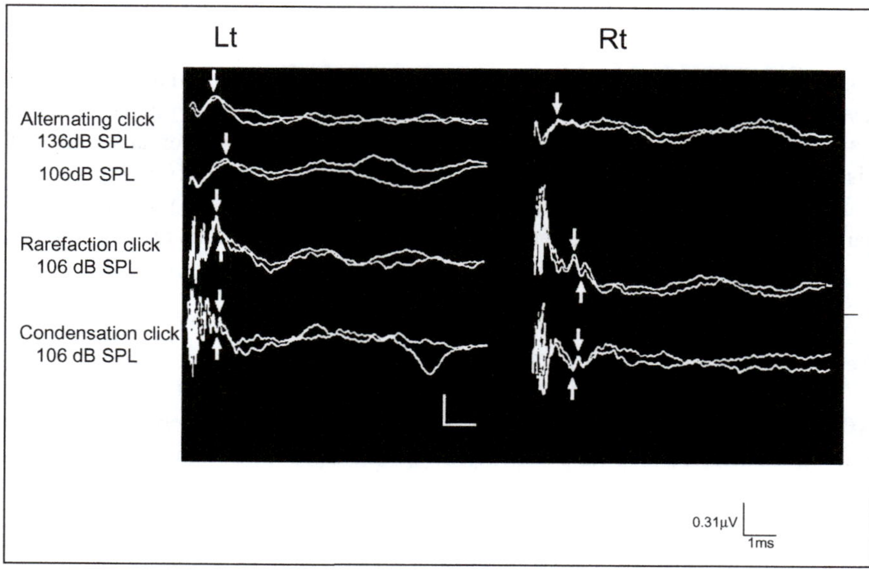

Fig. 2. Auditory brainstem response (ABR) of case 1. *Lt*, left; *Rt*, right; *arrows* indicate wave I

rarefaction clicks and was different with that induced by condensation clicks (Fig. 2) [11]. Distortion product otoacoustic emission (DPOAE) and transient evoked otoacoustic emissions (TEOAE) of otoacoustic emissions (OAE) were normal (Fig. 3). Electrocochleogram was normal (see Fig. 1).

Motor and sensory nerve conduction velocity (NCV) was completely normal with no signs of temporal dispersion.

Neuroimaging Examinations

T_1- and T_2-weighted cranial magnetic resonance imaging (MRI) showed no abnormal signal intensity.

We recommended to the patient and his family that he should be treated as a patient with auditory agnosia. He successfully entered a national school for the hearing impaired and now studies hard.

Case 2: Seven-Year-Old Girl

Her diagnosis is fluctuating hearing loss, episodic headache, and stroke with platelet hyperaggregability, with coexistence of auditory neuropathy and cochlear hearing loss [12].

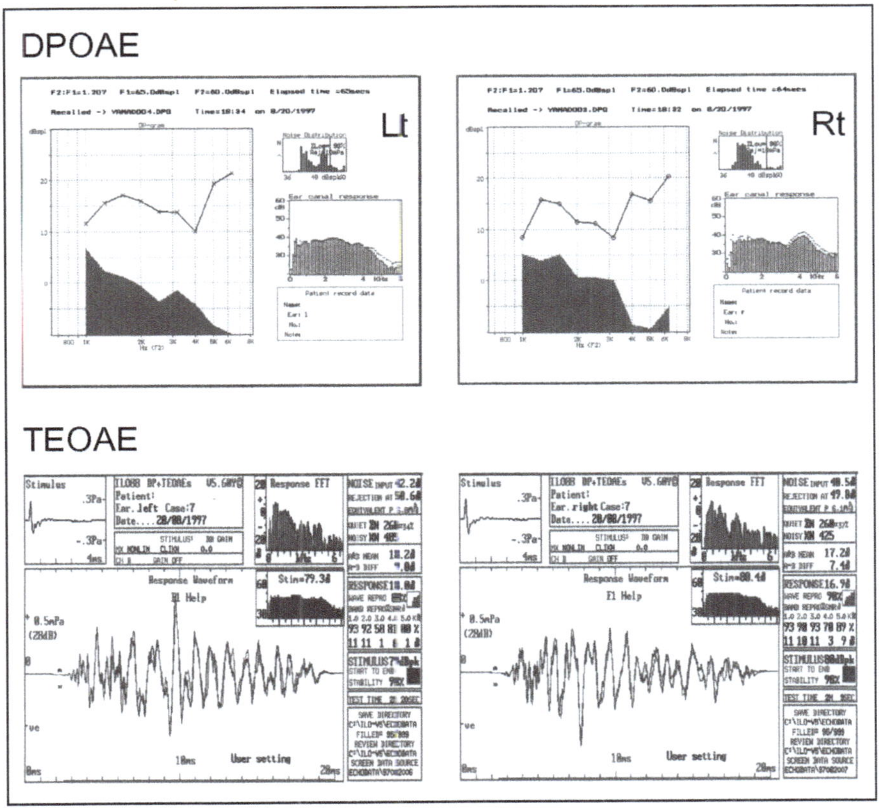

Fig. 3. Otoacoustic emission (OAE) of case 1. *Upper panels*, distortion product otoacoustic emission (DPOAE); *lower panels*, transient evoked otoacoustic emissions (TEOAE)

She was admitted to our hospital because of slowly progressive, fluctuating sensorineural hearing loss as well as episodic headache. She was born at 36 weeks of gestation after an uneventful pregnancy and delivery with birth weight of 1482 g. No asphyxia, hypoglycemia, or respiratory distress was evident at birth. Neonatal hyperbilirubinemia was appropriately treated by phototherapy. No medication was administered during her neonatal period. Family history was negative for neurological or hearing impairment and migraine. At 18 months of age, her parents first noted that she did not respond to their voices.

At the age of 3.8 years, during a febrile illness, the patient first manifested headache, vomiting, and dizziness. At the age of 4 years, bilateral hearing impairment worsened suddenly after prolonged running. Later, headaches and intermittent vertigo developed during viral infection, accompanied by deterioration of hearing. General physical and neurological findings during the attacks were normal.

At 5 years of age the patient began to use hearing aids. She continued to complain of episodic headaches over several years. General intellectual activity was normal. Hearing aids permitted her to communicate orally without difficulty. At 8 years of age, general physical and neurological examination was normal. Blood tests disclosed normal platelet counts with high titer of plasma thrombin–antithrombin III complex (TAT) (7.9 ng/ml; normal, 3.0). The platelet aggregation testing in vitro showed excessive aggregation in response to a low concentration of collagen. During a headache, the plasma TAT was 52.2 ng/ml, and the serum thromboxane (TX) B2, a metabolite of arachidonic acid, was slightly elevated. Then aspirin, ascorbic acid, and alpha-tocopherol acetate were administered to her. As platelet aggregability normalized, so did the plasma TAT concentration. Her headaches resolved.

Hearing Acuity and Auditory Perception

An audiometry at 3 years of age demonstrated hearing impairment that was most severe for higher frequencies (Fig. 4). Repeated audiometry showed gradual deterioration. We did not perform a word discrimination test; however, she could listen and talk with others without difficulty under condition of hearing amplification. She could understand environmental sounds.

Neurophysiological Findings

ABR indicated suspected left-sided cochlear microphonics with a threshold of 70 dB. On the right, ABR disclosed cochlear dysfunction with a threshold of

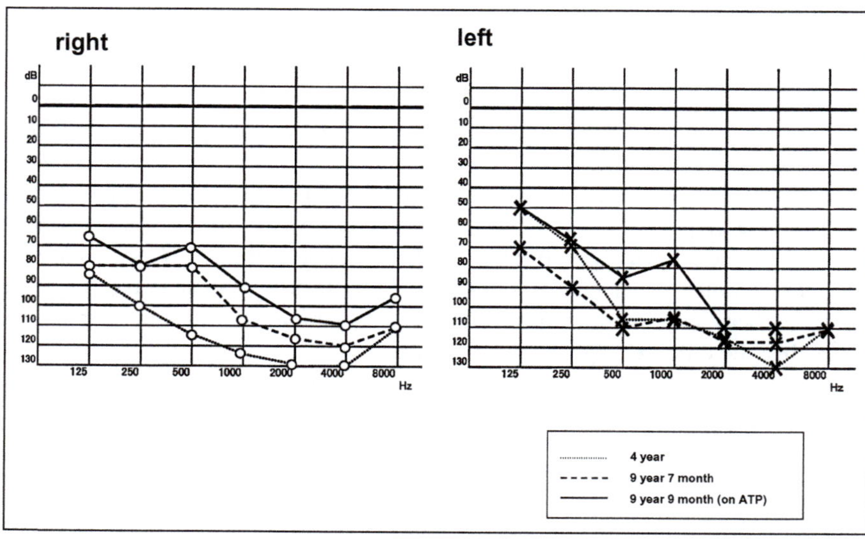

Fig. 4. Serial change of hearing in case 2

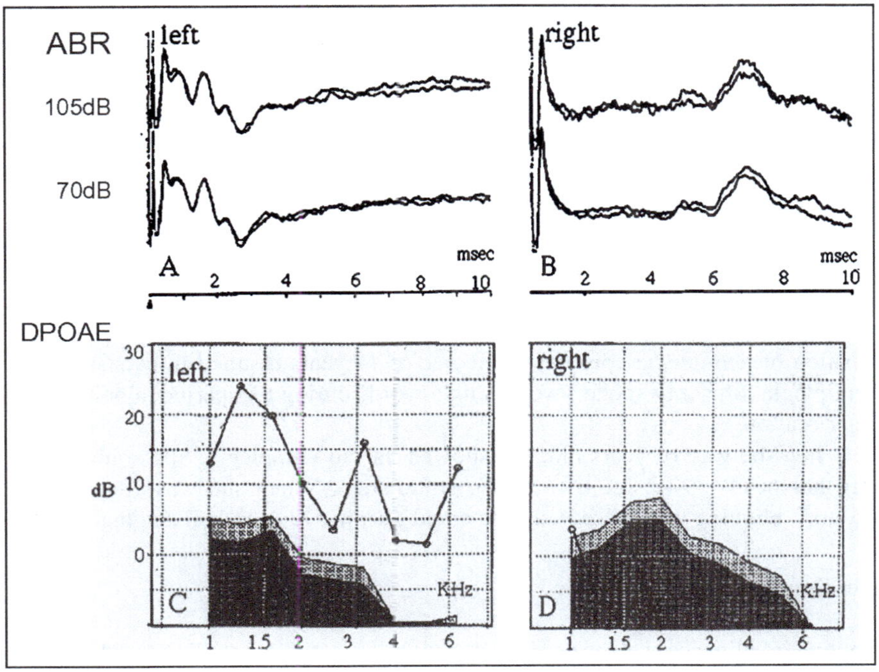

Fig. 5. ABR and DPOAE in case 2

105 dB (Fig. 5). DPOAE testing indicated damage to the outer hair cells in the right ear (see Fig. 4). NCVs were normal.

Neuroimaging Studies

Computed tomography (CT) at 3 years of age was normal. Brain MRI at 5 years of age showed bilateral multiple lesions of small infarction in cerebral white matter, whereas the brainstem appeared normal. After 18 months of aspirin and antioxidant therapy, no new white matter lesions could be found in subcortical or deep white matter by MRI.

This patient may have some similarity with Starr's patients reported in 1998 [13] in worsening with febrile diseases but has a difference in the accompanying disease.

Case 3: Sixteen-Year-Old Girl

Her diagnosis is alternating hemiplegia of childhood (AHC) with mental retardation and complex type of auditory neuropathy.

Detailed clinical history before the diagnosis of AN has been published elsewhere [14]. Her neurophysiological data were reported by Kon et al. [15].

She was born to unrelated healthy parents after a cesarean section because of placenta plevia. Tonic fits occurred 3 days after birth and were followed by abnormal ocular movements and generalized hypotonia. Episodic hemiplegia with preserved consciousness appeared at 1 year of age. Her psychomotor development was delayed. She spoke meaningful words at 2 years and 6 months of age.

Generalized seizures developed at 2 years of age. Thereafter, she had intractable epileptic seizures. In the ensuing years, both hemiplegic and generalized tonic seizure (GTS) episodes decreased with the use of medications including flunarizine to a few times a month for the former and a few times a year for the latter. Exacerbation of hemiplegic episodes at the age of 14 years resulted in persistent right hemiplegia. She only spoke several single words during this period, albeit without deterioration.

When she was 16 years old, she showed flaccid tetraplegia. She could weakly turn her head to the side of acoustic stimulation. When she was 18 years old, auditory blinking was preserved. She could turn her head to bell ringing.

Hearing and Cognitive Tests

Routine intelligence scale tests and subjective audiometry including word discrimination test could not be performed because she was too severely retarded.

Neurophysiological Findings

ABR was normal at 4 years of age, with a decreased waveform pattern at 16 years of age and absent ABR at 18 years of age. A DP-gram showed that all DP levels were higher than the noise floor levels, the range being 25 to 14 dB (Fig. 6). Total echo power (TEP) of TEOAE in the right and left ears were 8.1 and 7.3 dB, respectively. There were apparent response spectrum components from 0 ± 6 kHz bilaterally.

NCVs were normal.

Neuroimaging Studies

Brain CT at 10 years of age revealed mild cerebellar atrophy with vermian predominance.

Discussion

Auditory neuropathy (AN) or auditory nerve disease (AND) was first reported by different research groups in 1996 [1,2], although discrepancy of normal pure tone audiogram and ABR has rarely been noticed since the early days of ABR introduction to the clinical population [3–5]. However, this kind of clinical situation has not been fully understood as a noticeable entity until recently. Moreover, after common

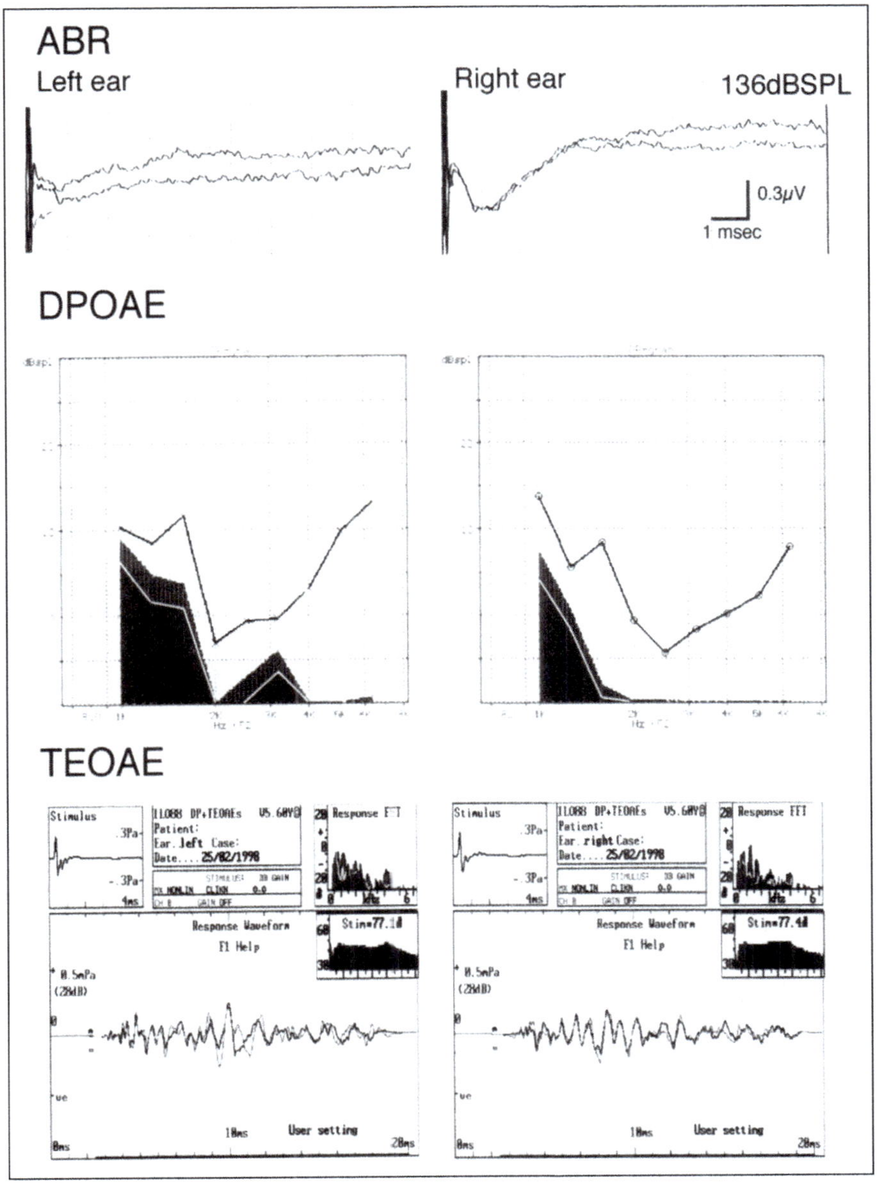

Fig. 6. ABR, DPOAE, and TEOAE of case 3

understanding of AN, the precise feature of auditory perception in patients with this pathological condition has not been described [16]. Then, the authors examined auditory perception in a patient with the pure type of AN and found the necessity of differential diagnosis with auditory verbal agnosia in this disorder [8,9].

Eight of ten AN patients in the work by Starr et al. in 1996 [4] showed neurological abnormalities including ataxic gait, weakness, and absent ankle jerk that suggested generalized neurological disease. Actually, three patients were diagnosed as having two types of CMTD. Two among the ten patients seemed to have the pure type of AN. Kaga et al. [5] reported the same category of two patients as AND. These patients were 53 and 68 years of age and had auditory and vestibular symptoms without apparent neurological symptoms such as CMTD.

In our patients, only one patient (case 1) was determined to have the pure type of AN. The other two cases had signs and symptoms of systemic neurological disease.

In case 1, ABR, OAE, and electrocochleogram (ECochG) showed typical findings of pure AN with no apparent underlying disease. He is now a college student, so the possibility of future CMTD or some type of hereditary sensory motor neuropathy (HSMN) in this patient seems to be decreasing. Clinical findings in this patient were very similar to central auditory processing disorder. Therefore, individual impairment in auditory perception should be clarified. This patient was finally diagnosed when he was 7 years old. The importance of both ABR and OAE examination in children with delayed speech is again noticed.

In case 2, the child's hearing deterioration was specific to her elevated body temperature, exercise, and viral infection. Her underlying pathophysiology was related to platelet aggregability, but her actual diagnosis is still pending decision. Hearing impairment and ABR/OAE abnormalities are surely compatible with AN.

In case 3, her intellectual level did not allow us to perform subjective tests for cognition and hearing. Limited objective tests of ABR and OAE demonstrated discrepancy of the results, which were compatible with AN. Moreover, her hearing was rather well preserved, which was revealed by her behavioral response. Her underlying disease was AHC. Its pathophysiology has not been clarified despite energetic exploration by many researchers for many years. A relationship with migraine and hemiplegia was sometimes mentioned [17] but was not proved in AHC.

Therefore, we would like to classify AN at least to two types. One is the "pure" type, and the other is the "complex" type in which AN is one of the symptoms of systemic disease. In the former type, AN cannot be ruled out as the first presenting symptom of the second type. However, from Starr's case, documentation [4] suggested that if the appropriate tests and systemic survey could be done at the appropriate time, classification of the two types seems not to be too difficult. In the previous article [18], we reported the pure type of AN as "an isolated and sporadic AN (AND)." Thus, we could propose AND for the pure type of AN and AN for the complex type, as the broad meanings of these pathophysiological states.

Recently, published reports on CMTD with and without AN stated an abnormal molecular basis [19] was clarified in some patients with AN. Moreover, cochlear implant is sometimes a candidate in AN. However, the results are various [20,21]. We should wait for an analysis of a large number of patients with the pure type of

AN, and it may be better to wait for established classification by more sophisticated methods such as gene study. However, from the clinical point of view, it is convenient to classify AN in these two types, pure or complex. Further, AN/AND as a clinical entity must be promoted more among personnel who take care of children with delayed speech and with childhood neurological diseases.

References

1. Worthington DW, Peters JF (1980) Quantifiable hearing and no ABR: paradox or error? Ear Hear 1:281–285
2. Kraus N, Ozdamar O, Stein L, et al (1984) Absent auditory brain stem response: peripheral hearing loss or brain stem dysfunction? Laryngoscope 94:400–406
3. Starr A, Picton TW, Sininger Y, et al (1996) Auditory neuropathy. Brain 119(pt 3):741–753
4. Deltenre P, Mansbach AL, Bozet C, et al (1997) Auditory neuropathy: a report on three cases with early onsets and major neonatal illnesses. Electroencephalogr Clin Neurophysiol 104:17–22
5. Kaga K, Nakamura M, Shinogami M, et al (1996) Auditory nerve disease of both ears revealed by auditory brainstem responses, electrocochleography and otoacoustic emissions. Scand Audiol 25:233–238
6. Rapin I, Gravel J (2003) "Auditory neuropathy": physiologic and pathologic evidence calls for more diagnostic specificity. Int J Pediatr Otorhinolaryngol 67:707–728
7. Kaga M, Kon K, Uno A, et al (2002) Auditory perception in auditory neuropathy: clinical similarity with auditory verbal agnosia. Brain Dev 24:197–202
8. Kaga M (1999) Language disorders in Landau–Kleffner syndrome. J Child Neurol 14: 118–122
9. Kaga M, Shindo M, Kaga K (2000) Long-term follow-up of auditory agnosia as a sequel of herpes encephalitis in a child. J Child Neurol 15:626–629
10. Kaga M (1992) Development of sound localization. Acta Paediatr Jpn 34:134–138
11. Berlin CI, Bordelon J, St John P, et al (1998) Reversing click polarity may uncover auditory neuropathy in infants. Ear Hear 19:37–47
12. Nobutoki T, Sasaki M, Fukumizu M, et al (2006) Fluctuating hearing loss, episodic headache, and stroke with platelet hyperaggregability: coexistence of auditory neuropathy and cochlear hearing loss. Brain Dev 28:55–59
13. Starr A, Sininger Y, Winter M, et al (1998) Transient deafness due to temperature-sensitive auditory neuropathy. Ear Hear 19:169–179
14. Saito Y, Sakurakawa N, Sasaki M, et al (1998) A case of alternating hemiplegia of childhood with cerebellar atrophy. Pediatr Neurol 19:65–68
15. Kon K, Inagaki M, Kaga M, et al (2000) Otoacoustic emission in patients with neurological disorders who have auditory brainstem response abnormality Brain Dev 22:327–335
16. Zeng FG, Oba S, Garde S, et al (1999) Temporal and speech processing deficits in auditory neuropathy. Neuroreport 10:3429–435
17. Shellhaas RA, Smith SE, O'Tool E, et al (2006) Mimics of childhood stroke: characteristics of a prospective cohort. Pediatrics 118:704–709
18. Sheykholeslami K, Kaga K, Kaga M (2001) An isolated and sporadic auditory neuropathy (auditory nerve disease): report of five patients. J Laryngol Otol 115:530–534
19. Butinar D, Starr A, J Zidar J, et al (2008) Auditory nerve is affected in one of two different point mutations of the neurofilament light gene. Clin Neurophysiol 119:367–375
20. Rance G, Beer DE, Cone-Wesson B, et al (1999). Clinical findings for a group of infants and young children with auditory neuropathy. Ear Hear 20:238–252
21. Walton J, Gibson WP, Sanli H, et al (2008) Predicting cochlear implant outcomes in children with auditory neuropathy. Otol Neurotol 29:302–309

A Case of Unilateral Auditory Neuropathy

Yuki Saito[1], Mitsuya Suzuki[2], and Tunemasa Sato[1]

Summary

We report a case of unilateral auditory neuropathy (AN) showing improvement in both pure tone hearing (PTA) and speech discrimination scores (SDS) with time. Some reports have documented the findings of auditory examination in patients with unilateral AN, and a few reports have documented the time-related changes in these findings for the same patients. A 3-year-old Japanese boy was referred to our hospital for audiological evaluation of his left ear. The audiogram showed normal hearing threshold in his right ear and severe sensorineural hearing loss in the left ear. DPOAE testing showed normal bilateral responses. ABR in the left ear showed no response of any waves in 110 dB hearing level, whereas the electrocochleogram (ECochG) showed broad compound action potentials (CAP) and the absence of N2. PTA and SDS at age 4 revealed slight improvement in the hearing threshold in the left ear.

Key words Auditory neuropathy, Unilateral, Electrocochleography

Introduction

Auditory neuropathy (AN), which is a syndrome found by Starr et al. [1], has been reported under different names such as auditory nerve disease [2] or essential retrocochlear lesions [3]. AN can be subdivided as to etiology into hereditary, a mix of etiologies including toxic and metabolic (anoxia, bilirubinemia), immunological (drug reaction, demyelination), and infectious (postviral). Idiopathic could be defined in almost 40% of affected individuals [4]. The classic criterion of AN first described by Starr et al. was a hearing impairment characterized by normal or near-normal pure tone hearing threshold with severe reduction of speech discrimination

[1]Department of Otolaryngology, Tokyo Metropolitan Police Hospital, 4-22-1 Nakano, Nakano-ku, Tokyo 164-8541, Japan
[2]Department of Otolaryngology, and Head and Neck Surgery, The University of Tokyo, Tokyo, Japan

doi: 10.1007/978-4-431-09433-3_14, © Springer 2009

score (SDS) [1]. Recently, this criterion has been changed to include patients who have severe elevation of pure tone hearing threshold [4]. Sininger and Starr [4] reported that 82% of the AN had symmetrical hearing loss, 14% had bilateral asymmetrical losses, and about 4% were unilateral hearing loss. We present a case of unilateral AN with improvement of both pure tone hearing and SDS with the passage of time.

Case Report

A 3-year-old Japanese boy was referred to our hospital for audiological evaluation in his left ear. He was born full term via normal spontaneous vaginal delivery without complications. Developmental milestones were acquired in an age-appropriate manner, including motor, coordination, and speech/language functions. He was in good health and was not taking any medications. There had been no episodes of ear infections or trauma. His mother noticed that he could not hear with his left ear. The family history had been unremarkable, but his grandmother might have unilateral deafness.

Pure tone audiometry, performed at age 3 years, revealed normal hearing sensitivity for his right ear and severe to profound sensorineural hearing loss for the left ear (Fig. 1). Normal speech recognition was evident for the right ear. Impedance audiometer recorded normal middle ear compliance bilaterally (type A tympanograms). The stapedial reflex in the left ear was elicited at appropriate sensation levels at all test frequencies by contralateral acoustic stimulation.

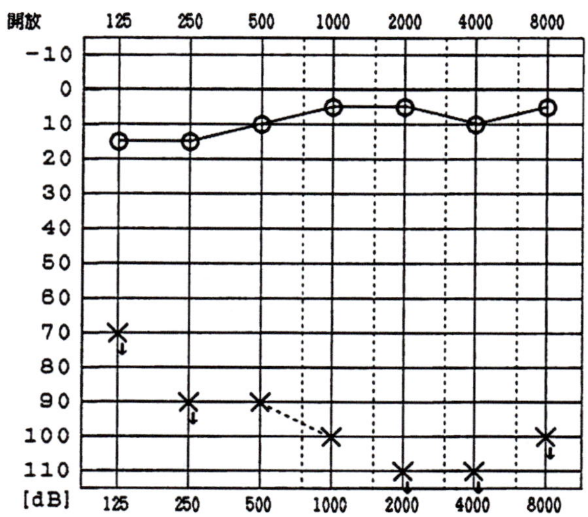

Fig. 1. Pure-tone audiometry of this patient on the first outpatient day showed normal hearing level for his right ear and severely disturbed hearing level for his left ear

Distortion-product otoacoustic emission (DPOAE) testing, which was performed at 1 to 8 kHz in each ear, using the ratio of $f_2/f_1 = 1.2$., showed normal bilateral responses, in spite of the degree of hearing loss (Fig. 2). Auditory evoked potentials (ABR) were performed at the 90 and 105 dB hearing level. ABR with 90 dB hearing level tracing for the right ear were characterized by clearly formed and repeatable wave peaks. Otherwise, ABR in the left ear showed no response of any waves at the 110 dB hearing level (Fig. 3). Vestibular evoked myogenic potential (VEMP) was recorded as normal response in bilateral ears. Computed tomography (CT) scan and magnetic resonance (MR) imaging showed normal internal auditory meatus and auditory nerve, but no acoustic tumor. Using the click stimulation, cochlear microphone was measured by pen-needle electrode put on the promontory under sedation (Fig. 4). The electrocochleogram (ECochG) showed broad compound action potentials (CAP) and the absence of N2.

We concluded that the left ear hearing loss is caused by AN and that the lesion may be between the inner hair cells and auditory nerve. In the pure tone audiometry performed at age 4, reduction of hearing threshold was observed in the left ear but not in the right ear (Fig. 5). DPOAE testing showed normal responses in both sides.

Discussion

AN can occur in isolation or in association with a peripheral neuropathy, for example, Charcot–Marie–Tooth disease, Friedreich's ataxia, Guillain–Barre syndrome, and multiple sclerosis. In case of Friedreich's ataxia and

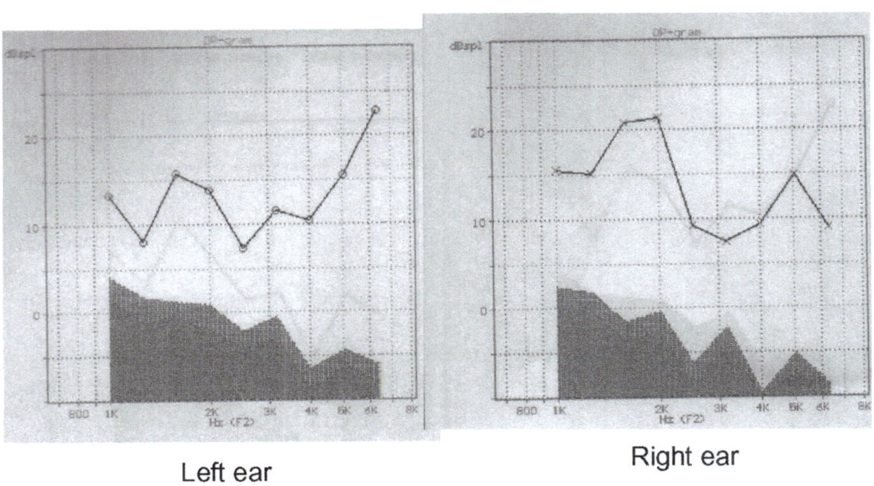

Fig. 2. Distortion-product otoacoustic emission (DPOAE) testing on the first outpatient day clearly showed normal response of the bilateral outer hair cell functions

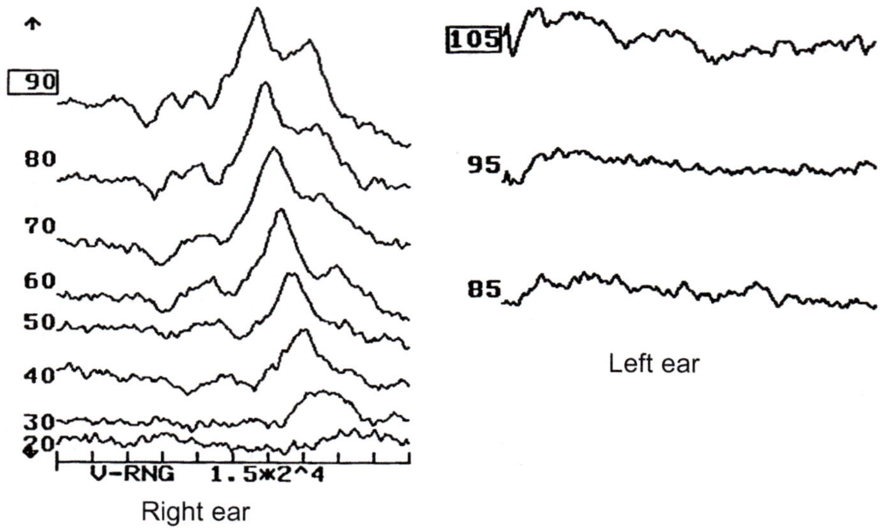

Fig. 3. Auditory evoked potential (ABR) of the patient showed quite normal response of his right ear and the loss of waves I to V of his left ear

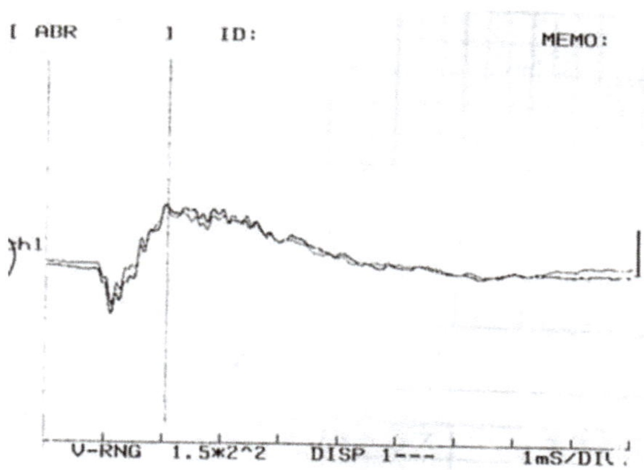

Fig. 4. Electrocochleography of the patient's left ear revealed a mild compound action potential (CAP) and loss of N2

Charcot–Marie–Tooth disease, postmortem examination has shown a degeneration of the spiral ganglion cells, which was either isolated or associated with a degeneration of the inner hair cells, or even demyelinization of the auditory nerve [5]. Thus, the hearing loss corresponds entirely to the general neurological disorder that is present in these patients. These cases showed slowly progressive hearing loss and did not benefit by amplification from hearing aids [1]. On the other

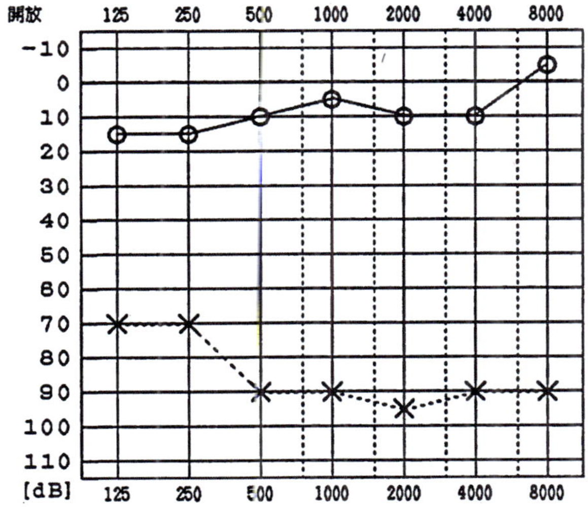

Fig. 5. Pure-tone audiogram at 4 years of age. Note the slightly improved hearing level of his left ear

hand, approximately two-thirds of the patients with AN have no evidence of concomitant peripheral neuropathy. A peripheral neuropathy was defined in approximately 80% of the subjects over 15 years of age. Thus, the association between AN and peripheral neuropathy is a common feature in adult but not young patients. Therefore, our patient must be carefully observed as he might experience peripheral neuropathy in the future. In addition, there may be alternative mechanisms (e.g., synaptic disorder or inner hair cell disorder) accounting for auditory nerve dysfunction.

The site of involvement of the auditory nerve in patients with AN is almost always in the distal segment because wave I of the ABR, which is generated within the temporal bone, is absent. Electrocochleography in AN patients was described in detail by Santarelli et al. [6]. A clearly identifiable CAP was found in the patient, but it took a rather broad morphology. These findings were likely to be the result of a reduced temporal synchrony of nerve fiber activation [3,4]. On the other hand, the absence of wave I of the ABR was quite noticeable. One possible explanation is that the nerve lesion was mainly localized in a more proximal portion with respect to the intracochlear segment, where CAP is believed to be generated. Moreover, Dauman et al. [7] reported that wave I could be generated by the eighth nerve at the medial part of the auditory internal meatus and, thus, more proximally with respect to the CAP source. The other possible explanation is that ABR, which is the far-field potential, could not record the desynchronized and low-amplitude postsynaptic potentials. On the other hand, CAP, which is the near-field potential, may be able to record the desynchronized and low-amplitude postsynaptic potentials [6].

Some reports have demonstrated findings of hearing examinations in patients with unilateral AN [8–12]. In addition, a few reports have demonstrated time-related change of hearing findings in those patients. Sininger and Starr [4] found that change of hearing loss caused by bilateral AN was usually fluctuating or progressing, rarely improving (Fig. 6). On the other hand, Madden et al. [13] reported that nine of bilateral AN showed improvement in behavioral thresholds over time, which indicated that a subset of children with AN may recover up to useful hearing levels. In our case, both pure tone hearing and SDS caused by unilateral AN have improved with the passage of time. It would be worth discussing whether the hearing improvement is the result of the patient's growth. It was suggested that the pure tone audiograms and SDS score improved in the affected ear with the passage of time because the threshold of the unaffected ear did not change.

Starr et al. [4] reported that the mean age of onset of auditory neuropathy symptoms is 9 years. Seventy-five percent of the patients were less than 10 years of age when symptoms were first seen. There is an approximately equal distribution of male and female patients with AN. Recently, AN has been found frequently in children, because automated ABR has spread worldwide as hearing screening in newborns. Rance et al. [14] reported that 0.23% of the infants at high risk for hearing impairment had AN; therefore, AN would be more common in the infant population than previously suspected. Sininger and Starr [4] reported that the 59 patients included 2 years old or younger 25 AN patients, who may be associated with hyperbilirubinemia and prematurity. For our patient, the episode of such a high risk did not happen in either the newborn or the infant period. As our patient did not undergo hearing screening with automated ABR as a newborn, it is uncertain whether unilateral AN in this case is acquired or congenital.

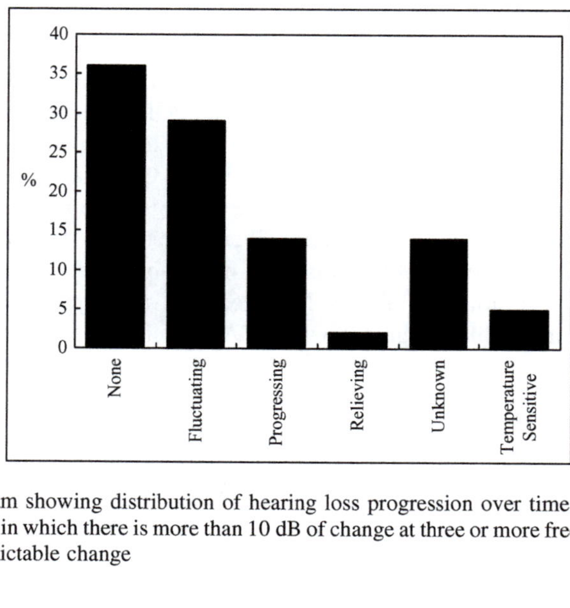

Fig. 6. Histogram showing distribution of hearing loss progression over time. Fluctuating loss is defined as that in which there is more than 10 dB of change at three or more frequencies between tests but no predictable change

References

1. Starr A, Picton TW, Sininger Y, et al (1996) Auditory neuropathy. Brain 119:741–753
2. Kaga K, Nakamura M, Shinogami M, et al (1996) Auditory nerve disease of both ears revealed by auditory brainstem responses, electrocochleography and otoacoustic emissions. Scand Audiol 25:233–238
3. Satoh T, Suzuki H, Yahata N (1985) Audiological findings in patients with essential retrocochlear lesions. Audiol Jpn 28:758–771 (in Japanese)
4. Sininger Y, Starr A (2001) Auditory neuropathy, a new perspective on hearing disorders. Singular, San Diego, CA, pp 1–13
5. Spoendling H (1974) Optic and cochleovestibular degenerations in hereditary ataxias: II. Temporal bone pathology in two cases of Friedreich's ataxia with vestibulo-cochlear disorders. Brain 97:41–48
6. Santarelli R, Arslan E (2002) Electrocochleography in auditory neuropathy. Hear Res 170:32–47
7. Dauman R, Aran JM, Portmann M (1988) Limits of ABR and contribution of transtympanic electrocochleography in the assessment of cerebellopontine angle tumours. Clin Otolaryngol Allied Sci 13:107–114
8. Jerger J, Ali A, Fong K, et al (1992) Otoacoustic emissions, audiometric sensitivity loss, and speech understanding: a case study. J Am Acad Audiol 3:283–286
9. Konradsson KS (1996) Bilaterally preserved otoacoustic emissions in four children with profound idiopathic unilateral sensorineural hearing loss. Audiology 35:217–227
10. Kothe C, Fleischer S, Breitfuss A (2006) Unilateral auditory neuropathy. A rare differential diagnosis of unilateral deafness. HNO 54:215–220 (in German)
11. Wang D, Bu X, Li X, et al (2005) Study of unilateral auditory neuropathy in infants. Lin Chuang Er Bi Yan Hou Ke Za Zhi 19:729–732 (in Chinese)
12. Podwall A, Podwall D, Gordon TG, et al (2002) Unilateral auditory neuropathy: case study. J Child Neurol 17:306–309
13. Madden C, Rutter M, Lisa Hilbert, et al (2002) Clinical and audiological features in auditory neuropathy. Arch Otolaryngol Head Neck Surg 128:1026–1030
14. Rance G, Beer DE, Cone-Wesson B, et al (1999) Clinical findings for a group of infants and young children with auditory neuropathy. Ear Hear 20:238–252

Part VI
Historical Issues

Prehistory of Auditory Neuropathy in Japan

Toshihiro Tsuzuku

Summary

Briefly, I describe the research history of auditory neuropathy in Japan. Researchers of audiology in Japan had almost established the concept of this disease before the 1980s. Until that time, the previous researchers in Japan were educated in German medicine and found it difficult to publish in English. For example, this language problem is exemplified by the question as to who is the first to describe endolymphatic hydrops of Meniere's disease. Prof. Kowashiro Yamakawa, who was professor of otolaryngology at the Osaka Imperial University, reported the world's first case of inner ear histopathology of that disease, in German, in 1935. Hallpike et al. reported the second case in 1936, in English. Although the bibliography worldwide has long regarded Hallpike's work as the first report of Meniere's disease, I wish to report the historical fact of auditory neuropathy, of which pathophysiology was firstly described in Japanese.

Key words Auditory neuropathy, Meniere's disease, Japan

Introduction

The aim of this short report is to describe the research history in Japan of auditory neuropathy before 1996. From this history you can understand that development of technology in audiology is closely related to clarification of the pathophysiology of this disease.

Department of Otolaryngology, Teikyo University School of Medicine, 2-11-1 Kaga, Itabashi-ku, Tokyo 173-8605, Japan

doi: 10.1007/978-4-431-09433-3_15,

The Age of Establishing Speech Audiometry

After the pure tone audiometer was introduced in audiological psychology, the speech audiometry was established. In Japan, in the 1950s, an otolaryngologist who paid attention to audiology developed the speech audiometry, which is widely used in ORL clinics.

Afterwards, some otologists noticed that there were patients who complained of poor speech discrimination, in contrast to the results of pure tone audiometry, without any retrocochlear lesions. In 1955, Kunio Arai [1] reported these cases, and proposed a new concept of hearing loss: he named this disease bilateral retrocochlear hearing loss. He speculated that the lesion should be located at the auditory pathway from the cochlear nerve to brainstem and suggested there might be degeneration of the nerve.

The Age of Discovering ECochG and ABR

In the 1970s, electrophysiological research in audiology was advanced by using the newly discovered techniques of the electrocochleogram (ECochG) and auditory brainstem response (ABR). A Japanese physician in audiology, Dr. Tumemasa Sato, reported these cases with the results of ECochG and ABR and proposed a new concept of the disease. In 1985, he published his work in *Audiology Japan* (in Japanese) and named this disease as idiopathic retrocochlear hearing loss [2]. He summarized the clinical features of this disease as below:

- Bilateral hearing loss; it occurs at adolescence
- Variant audiogram; mild hearing thresholds elevation
- Speech discrimination shows as worse compared to pure tone hearing threshold
- Difficult to detect sound localization
- ABR shows flat wave and no peak
- ECochG shows low amplitudes and broad summating potential (SP)
- Normal functions of vestibular system
- Computed tomography (CT) scan of head and EEG show normal results

Sato speculated that the lesion should exist in the retrocochlear auditory pathway from the results of poor speech discrimination, as reported by Kaga. His speculation of the results of ECochG and ABR was described next. ABR is a far-field potential, and wave I of ABR is generated from the cochlear nerve. Absence of wave I means difficulty in electrical synchronization of the nerve itself. The SP is originated from the cochlea; thus, it should be normal cochlear function. Then, he concluded the lesion should be located in the cochlear nerve and suggested the pathogenesis might be neural degeneration.

The starting point of these studies was the discrepancy of the results between speech discrimination and pure tone hearing threshold. Therefore, the cases were all adults, and there was little knowledge about their vestibular function. The transient otoacoustic emissions (TOAE) and distortion product OAE (DPOAE) were introduced in the next decade. Nowadays, ear, nose, and throat (ENT) doctors and audiologists tend to diagnose the patients as having auditory neuropathy from only the results of ABR and TOAE or DPOAE testing. We should not forget the nature of this disease is poor speech discrimination.

References

1. Arai K (1955) Speech discrimination in cases of retro-cochlear hearing loss. Jiko 27:673–677 (in Japanese)
2. Sato T, Suzuki H, Yawata N, et al (1985) Hearing ability in cases of retro-cochlear hearing loss. Audiol Jpn 28:758–771 (in Japanese)

Is Auditory Neuropathy an Appropriate Diagnosis if There Is No Neuropathy?

Roger R. Marsh[1,2] **and Ken Kazahaya**[2,3]

Summary

In the initial reports of auditory neuropathy, there was ample evidence that the patients did indeed have neuropathy—a disease or disorder of the auditory nerve or other peripheral nerves. In the years that followed, the diagnosis has been applied to all cases in which the cochlear microphonic potentials or otoacoustic emissions were present and the auditory brainstem response absent, whether or not the nerve was known to be affected. At one time an argument could have been made that the lesion could be presumed to be in the auditory nerve because it was not proven that selective inner hair cell impairment even existed as a clinical entity. It has become clear, however, that mutations of the OTOF gene, and perhaps other genes, can cause a defect of inner hair cell function that is quite different from a true neuropathy. These patients differ from those with neuropathy in age of onset, severity of loss, prognosis, and often in potential for benefit from cochlear implantation. The time has come to reserve the diagnosis of auditory neuropathy for those cases in which there is evidence of a disorder of the auditory nerve.

Key words Auditory neuropathy, Cochlear implantation, Otoferlin, Inner hair cell, Otoacoustic emissions

Introduction

The landmark reports by Starr [1] and Kaga [2] and their colleagues introduced the medical and audiological communities to the concept of auditory neuropathy (AN), a disorder of the peripheral auditory nerve. These articles are best known for

[1]Center for Childhood Communication, and [2]Division of Pediatric Otolaryngology, The Children's Hospital of Philadelphia, 324 S. 34th Street, Philadelphia, PA 19104, USA

[3]Department of Otolaryngology: Head and Neck Surgery, University of Pennsylvania School of Medicine, Philadelphia, PA, USA

doi: 10.1007/978-4-431-09433-3_16,

demonstrating the diagnostic power of physiological tests [it is tempting to say "electrophysiological tests," but the otoacoustic emission (OAE) signal is not electric]; most of the cases had present cochlear microphonic potentials (CMs) or OAEs but absent auditory brainstem (ABR) responses. It is often forgotten, however, that each report cited other evidence for neuropathy. In the years that followed, many clinicians have applied the diagnosis of AN to virtually any case having the requisite ABR, OAE, and CM findings, whether or not there was independent evidence of nerve involvement.

At one time, an argument might have been made for such diagnoses. The only alternative to neuropathy with these physiological findings is impairment of the inner hair cells (IHCs), with preservation of the outer hair cells (OHCs). There were almost no reports in the literature of selective IHC loss in humans—none in which there was adequate physiological testing. But even as evidence appeared that IHC function could be impaired without substantial loss of auditory nerve fibers or even of the hair cells themselves, the diagnosis of AN was applied to cases of proven IHC impairment.

This imprecision in terminology is no longer justified. It causes confusion and obscures the literature. It gives rise to the nonsensical conclusion that selective impairment of IHCs is AN, but the same IHC impairment, with impairment of OHCs, is not. The time has come to reserve the diagnosis of AN for those cases in which there is evidence—clinical, genetic, or perhaps in the future electrophysiological—that the auditory nerve is involved.

A Concise History

Although the term neuropathy can be applied to any disease or disorder of any nerve, it is most commonly applied to disorders of the peripheral nervous system, including peripheral portions of nerves with their cell bodies in the central nervous system (CNS). Although some disorders have both peripheral and central effects, the distinction between central and peripheral is not arbitrary. Many of the neuropathies involve defects of myelination, as do many encephalopathies—disorders of nerves within the brain. In the periphery, myelin arises from Schwann cells, whereas in the CNS the oligodendrocytes are responsible. Each cell type is susceptible to different genetic disorders. There are nongenetic neuropathies as well, but here too there is differential susceptibility. Not all neuropathies primarily target the myelin or are confined to the myelin. There can be loss of axons or even cell death. The manifestations of neuropathy are varied. In demyelination, nerve conduction is slowed, but there can also be partial or complete block; a neuron might be unable to initiate or propagate a nerve impulse, or initiation may require an intense stimulus. Symptoms can be sensory, motor, or both. Often, but not always, nerves serving the legs are most affected, because the length of the axon increases susceptibility.

It has long been known that hearing loss can be a feature of certain neuropathies. The classic example is Friedreich's ataxia, a disorder in which the axons, and ultimately the cell bodies, of large myelinated nerves die. There can be auditory and vestibular involvement. Spoendlin's classic 1974 treatise [3] describes the temporal bone findings in two sisters. Both had extensive loss of spiral ganglion cells, one sister having nearly complete loss, and the other having a nearly normal complement in the hook of the base, with increasing loss toward the apex. Both had substantial loss of vestibular nerves in the ampullar branch, with less in the branches serving the utricle and saccule. One set of cochleas had extensive postmortem changes, but in the other survival of IHCs and OHCs was evident. Friedreich's ataxia was among the first of the neuropathies to be studied systematically by ABR [4]. Even in cases with normal or nearly normal pure tone thresholds, the ABR is often absent.

Long before the term AN was introduced, there had been reports of hearing loss in other neuropathies, notably the hereditary motor and sensory neuropathies (HMSNs) known as Charcot–Marie–Tooth disease [5,6]. The HMSNs are a heterogeneous group with more than two dozen types and subtypes, differing by symptoms, histological findings, mode of inheritance, and responsible mutation. Symptoms appear most often in the legs, with hearing loss being uncommon in most types. The early ABR reports noted prolongation of the interval between the peaks of waves I and III in many cases, consistent with demyelination; absence of all waves was uncommon [7,8].

Not all neuropathies are hereditary. Viruses, autoimmune disease, diabetes, and toxins can attack the peripheral nerves. One neuropathy, which few of the readers will encounter, seems often to be associated with hearing impairment. Cassava root, a staple food in much of the tropics, contains a compound that produces cyanide if the root is not properly prepared. Chronic cyanide toxicity, in combination with malnutrition, is suspected in tropical ataxic neuropathy, a significant public health problem in some parts of the world. In one exhaustive survey of an affected community in Nigeria, the disease was found in 7.7% of those screened [9]. Of the affected individuals, 16% had bilateral sensorineural hearing loss. There are no reports of ABR testing in this disorder.

The Diagnosis of AN

Although hearing loss was long known to be associated with neuropathies, it has in the past been classified as sensorineural, a term then used for nearly any hearing loss that was neither conductive nor caused by retrocochlear tumors. Indeed, many still refer to sensory losses as sensorineural, even in cases where the lesion is known to be at the level of the hair cells. In 1996, Starr and colleagues [1] brought attention to AN as a distinct entity. Ten cases were described. The ABR was absent in nine cases, and abnormal in one, a small wave V being identifiable only with high-intensity clicks in spite of only mild hearing loss. OAEs were present in all cases.

It is noteworthy that the diagnosis of AN was not made simply on the basis of the ABR and OAE findings. In eight cases, other signs of neuropathy were found. Most cases had several other features in common: mild to moderate bilateral hearing impairment, speech recognition scores much worse than would be expected for a sensory loss, and an age of onset—mid-childhood to early adulthood—similar to that of many neuropathies. Starr and colleagues recognized that that ABR and OAE findings did not themselves place the lesion at the level of the auditory nerve, but inferred the site of lesion from the combination of auditory and other tests and the clinical findings, as well as evidence of auditory nerve involvement in earlier reports of neuropathy.

Also in 1996, a report by Kaga et al. [2] provided corroboration, describing two cases in which ABRs were absent but OAEs and CMs were present. The affected patients had only mild threshold elevation but remarkably poor word recognition. Both had vestibular deficits. Kaga and colleagues had the misfortune to label the condition as auditory nerve disease—precisely the same diagnosis as AN, but not the term that caught the attention of the audiological and otological community.

Is It Neuropathy?

The rigor of the Starr and Kaga reports in making the diagnosis of AN is lacking from many subsequent reports in the literature. Indeed it became common to make the diagnosis solely on the basis of absence of ABR and presence of OAEs or CMs, without regard to other evidence of neuropathy [10–12]. Starr and colleagues had recognized from the start that the physiological tests did not differentiate true neuropathy from IHC disorders, but argued as recently as 2001 that such IHC disorders had not been identified in hearing-impaired individuals [13,14].

Others had expressed concern about the use of the AN diagnosis. In 2001, Amatuzzi and colleagues published a report of histological examinations of the temporal bones of 15 deceased patients of a neonatal intensive care unit (NICU) [15]. In 3 cases, there was selective loss of IHCs. Each infant had died before 1 month of age after a stormy perinatal course. In none of the 15 pairs of cochleas was there obvious loss of neurons. The authors argued that their data suggest IHC loss as an alternative to auditory nerve disorder in cases with absent ABR and present OAEs. Their hypothesis certainly deserves consideration in the diagnosis of hearing impairment in NICU graduates, but it was a bit harsh to characterize the 1996 Starr [1] cases as having a postulated "theoretical auditory neuropathy," considering the mass of collaborating clinical data that Starr et al. had marshaled. The Amatuzzi article itself is far from conclusive. Although each of the 3 infants had failed ABR screening at least once in each ear, that is hardly evidence of absence of ABRs. Because screening was performed at 40 dB nHL, failure might reflect a conductive impairment. Even infants with normal peripheral auditory systems may fail because of poor recording conditions or because of damage to the brainstem auditory pathways; the screening device that was used does not record wave I and does not save waveforms for visual inspection. Would the loss of IHCs even have abolished the ABR? In most of the cochleas there was less than 50% loss of IHCs, quite possibly leaving enough survivors to generate an ABR.

Berlin et al. also have argued against the uncritical application of the AN diagnosis [16]. A part of their argument was semantic, that the AN label discouraged cochlear implantation, but Berlin also noted the Amatuzzi report and the many patients in his series who had no reported signs of neuropathy. Unfortunately, Berlin's proposal, to use the term auditory dys-synchrony as a supplement or replacement for AN, is less than satisfactory. Marsh [17] responded that disordered synchrony of neural discharge is only one facet of AN; there can be cell death or conduction block as well, and dys-synchrony cannot account for threshold elevation. Furthermore, IHC impairment would not cause dys-synchrony. Rapin and Gravel have cautioned against the casual diagnosis of AN, citing concerns about the imprecision of the term when the lesion is not in the auditory nerve [18,19]. They appear to emphasize the need to differentiate AN from central involvement, for example, the cochlear nucleus in hyperbilirubinemia, but the astute clinician should be able to make that differential diagnosis by observing the presence or absence of wave I in the ABR.

Two lines of investigation have fundamentally changed the debate. Investigators have thoroughly characterized families in whom HMSN is commonly associated with hearing impairment, leaving no doubt that AN, as originally described by Starr, is a legitimate clinical diagnosis [20]. One report is exemplary [21]. In a single family, HMSN and AN are traced through three generations. Clinical and physiological findings of audiological and neurological status are presented. The responsible gene and even the mutation within the gene are identified. Finally, temporal bone histology is presented for a deceased affected family member. The organ of Corti was normal, but there was 95% loss of auditory neurons, and the axons of the few survivors demonstrated aberrant remyelination. It appears that not all AN is the result of demyelination or axonopathy. In the 1996 article, Starr and colleagues had hypothesized that the lesion could be at the level of the dendrites. Indeed, there may be such an AN. In DFNA9, a progressive deafness caused by mutation of the COCH gene, there appears to be deposition of a substance in the channels through which the dendrites of the auditory and vestibular nerve pass, strangling them [22]. There is also some loss of cell bodies and axons, but affected individuals do well with cochlear implants.

However, evidence has also accumulated that makes a clear and convincing case for IHC impairment in certain cases of so-called AN. In 1999, Yasunaga and colleagues identified the OTOF gene and published a thorough description of the gene's function and of the effect of a mutation of the gene [23]. The gene was identified through genetic analysis of four unrelated consanguineous families in Lebanon, in whom there were multiple cases of severe to profound prelingual sensorineural hearing impairment. The gene's role in deafness was verified when a specific mutation was found in 30 affected individuals but not in unaffected Lebanese controls. Analysis of the gene suggested that the protein it encoded, otoferlin, is involved in fusion of synaptic vesicles to the cell membrane, the essential step for release of transmitter substance in the synapse. Animal studies showed high OTOF activity in the IHCs but not elsewhere in the cochlea. Of note, the IHCs are grossly intact, hence the failure of temporal bone studies to reveal inner hair cell deafness. It can be speculated that the survival of the hair cells, even without functioning synapses, might contribute to nerve survival through release of trophic factors. Other researchers have examined the role of otoferlin in the release of transmitter from the IHC [24]. There is ample confirmation that ABRs are absent but OAEs are most often present in DFNB9, the deafness caused by OTOF mutations [11,25]. Affected children who receive cochlear implants are reported to do well [26]. Robust electrically elicited ABR or eighth-nerve action potentials can be recorded when the nerve is stimulated by the implant, confirming good nerve survival. Remarkably many authors refer to DFNB9 as AN; in the otoferlin literature, it appears that only Loundon et al. [27] argue that the term should be reserved for cases of true neuropathy.

What's in a Name?

Perhaps "a rose by any other name would smell as sweet," but telling someone to "Send a dozen red sausages to my sweetheart" would most likely cause confusion. Diagnosing AN without regard to evidence of neuropathy or in spite of evidence of IHC dysfunction is no less confusing and may have more serious consequences. Consider the literature on cochlear implantation in AN. The report by Shallop and colleagues [10], on cochlear implantation of five children with AN, has been cited again and again as evidence that implants are effective in this disorder, but there is no independent evidence of neuropathy. To the contrary, the cases seem to be more consistent with the descriptions of DFNB9, the deafness caused by IHC impairment. All had severe to profound hearing impairment of prelingual onset. None had other neurological findings.

Now that IHC impairment is a proven entity, it is especially egregious to call such cases AN. Consider this: Clinically, IHC impairment is indistinguishable from other cases of profound sensory deafness. They differ only in the presence of useless OHCs. Also, IHC deafness differs clinically from true neuropathy in many ways: site of lesion, residual hearing, age of onset in the case of HMSN or etiology in the case of suspected AN in NICU babies, survival or stimulability of the auditory nerve in the case of Friedreich's ataxia and perhaps in some HMSNs. Almost all that the IHC defect has in common with AN are the ABR and OAE or CM findings.

What shall we do? Why not reserve the diagnosis of AN for cases in which there is evidence of a true neuropathy? The evidence might be circumstantial—an age of onset, pure tone audiogram, and speech recognition scores typical of HMSN with AN. A presumptive diagnosis might be made if there are confirmed cases among siblings. More direct evidence might be available in some cases, such as neurological signs of neuropathy or results of genetic testing. Keep in mind, also, that ABRs need not be absent in auditory neuropathy; prolongation of the I–III interval, without obliteration of the ABR, has been reported in HMSN, suggesting involvement of the auditory nerve [7,8,28].

What about unilateral auditory neuropathy? Caution is advised. Absent ABR with preservation of OAEs in congenital unilateral profound impairment is more likely to reflect agenesis of the auditory nerve [29].

In cases of IHC impairment, the diagnosis should be sensory hearing loss. At the same time, clinicians would do well to abandon sensorineural loss in other cases, such as moderate loss with recruitment, which can confidently be diagnosed as sensory.

There remain areas of uncertainty. Many of the individuals said to have AN are NICU graduates. Hyperbilirubinemia has been implicated, but these infants have often suffered many other insults during their difficult perinatal courses. As already discussed, the report of Amatuzzi et al. [15] points to IHCs, but Rapin and Gravel [18,19] suspect the cochlear nucleus. Until new tests can resolve the issue or long-term follow-up can identify AN-like audiological results, or temporal bones become available for study, we must diagnose the cases as we always have, as sensorineural hearing loss, noting the atypical findings and uncertain prognosis.

References

1. Starr A, Picton TW, Sininger Y, et al (1996) Auditory neuropathy. Brain 119:741–753
2. Kaga K, Nakamura M, Shinogami M, et al (1996) Auditory nerve disease of both ears revealed by auditory brainstem responses, electrocochleography and otoacoustic emissions. Scand Audiol 25:233–238
3. Spoendlin H (1974) Optic cochleovestibular degenerations in hereditary ataxias. II. Temporal bone pathology in two cases of Friedreich's ataxia with vestibulo-cochlear disorders. Brain 97:41–48
4. Satya-Murti S, Cacace A, Hanson P (1980) Auditory dysfunction in Friedreich ataxia: result of spiral ganglion degeneration. Neurology 30:1047–1053
5. Cornell J, Sellars S, Beighton P (1984) Autosomal recessive inheritance of Charcot-Marie-Tooth disease associated with sensorineural deafness. Clin Genet 25:163–165
6. Musiek FE, Weider DJ, Mueller RJ (1982) Audiologic findings in Charcot-Marie-Tooth disease. Arch Otolaryngol 108:595–599
7. Kowalski JW, Rasheva M, Zakrzewska B (1991) Visual and brainstem auditory evoked potentials in hereditary motor-sensory neuropathy. Electromyogr Clin Neurophysiol 31:167–172
8. Garg BP, Markand ON, Bustion PF (1982) Brainstem auditory evoked responses in hereditary motor-sensory neuropathy: site of origin of wave II. Neurology 32:1017–1019
9. Oluwole OS, Onabolu AO, Link H, et al (2000) Persistence of tropical ataxic neuropathy in a Nigerian community. J Neurol Neurosurg Psychiatry 69:96–101
10. Shallop JK, Peterson A, Facer GW, et al (2001) Cochlear implants in five cases of auditory neuropathy: postoperative findings and progress. Laryngoscope 111:555–562
11. Rodriguez-Ballesteros M, del Castillo FJ, Martin Y, et al (2003) Auditory neuropathy in patients carrying mutations in the otoferlin gene (OTOF). Hum Mutat 22:451–456

12. Trautwein PG, Sininger YS, Nelson R (2000) Cochlear implantation of auditory neuropathy. J Am Acad Audiol 11:309–315
13. Sininger Y, Oba S (2001) Patients with auditory neuropathy: who are they and what can they hear? In: Sininger Y, Starr A (eds) Auditory neuropathy: a new perspective on hearing disorders. Singular, San Diego, pp 15–35
14. Starr A, Sininger Y, Nguyen T, et al (2001) Cochlear receptor (microphonic and summating potentials, otoacoustic emissions) and auditory pathway (auditory brain stem potentials) activity in auditory neuropathy. Ear Hear 22:91–99
15. Amatuzzi MG, Northrop C, Liberman MC, et al (2001) Selective inner hair cell loss in premature infants and cochlea pathological patterns from neonatal intensive care unit autopsies. Arch Otolaryngol Head Neck Surg 127:629–636
16. Berlin C, Hood L, Rose K (2001) On renaming auditory neuropathy as auditory dys-synchrony. Audiol Today 13(6):15–17
17. Marsh RR (2002) Is it auditory dys-synchrony? Comment on "On renaming auditory neuropathy as auditory dys-synchrony." Audiol Today 14(3):36–37
18. Rapin I, Gravel JS (2006) Auditory neuropathy: a biologically inappropriate label unless acoustic nerve involvement is documented. J Am Acad Audiol 17:147–150
19. Rapin I, Gravel J (2003) "Auditory neuropathy": physiologic and pathologic evidence calls for more diagnostic specificity. Int J Pediatr Otorhinolaryngol 67:707–728
20. Butinar D, Zidar J, Leonardis L, et al (1999) Hereditary auditory, vestibular, motor, and sensory neuropathy in a Slovenian Roma (Gypsy) kindred. Ann Neurol 46:36–44
21. Starr A, Michalewski HJ, Zeng FG, et al (2003) Pathology and physiology of auditory neuropathy with a novel mutation in the MPZ gene (Tyr145→Ser). Brain 126:1604–1619
22. Vermeire K, Brokx JP, Wuyts FL, et al (2006) Good speech recognition and quality-of-life scores after cochlear implantation in patients with DFNA9. Otol Neurotol 27:44–49
23. Yasunaga S, Grati M, Cohen-Salmon M, et al (1999) A mutation in OTOF, encoding otoferlin, a FER-1-like protein, causes DFNB9, a nonsyndromic form of deafness. Nat Genet 21:363–369
24. Roux I, Safieddine S, Nouvian R, Grati M, et al (2006) Otoferlin, defective in a human deafness form, is essential for exocytosis at the auditory ribbon synapse. Cell 20(127):277–289
25. Varga R, Kelley PM, Keats BJ, et al (2003) Non-syndromic recessive auditory neuropathy is the result of mutations in the otoferlin (OTOF) gene. J Med Genet 40:45–50
26. Rouillon I, Marcolla A, Roux I, et al (2006) Results of cochlear implantation in two children with mutations in the OTOF gene. Int J Pediatr Otorhinolaryngol 70:689–696
27. Loundon N, Marcolla A, Roux I, et al (2005) Auditory neuropathy or endocochlear hearing loss? Otol Neurotol 26:748–754
28. Guergueltcheva V, Tournev I, Bojinova V, et al (2006) Early clinical and electrophysiologic features of the two most common autosomal recessive forms of Charcot-Marie-Tooth disease in the Roma (Gypsies). J Child Neurol 21:20–25
29. Buchman CA, Roush PA, Teagle HF, et al (2006) Auditory neuropathy characteristics in children with cochlear nerve deficiency. Ear Hear 27:399–408

Subject Index

GPSR Compliance

The European Union's (EU) General Product Safety Regulation (GPSR) is a set of rules that requires consumer products to be safe and our obligations to ensure this.

If you have any concerns about our products, you can contact us on ProductSafety@springernature.com

In case Publisher is established outside the EU, the EU authorized representative is:

Springer Nature Customer Service Center GmbH
Europaplatz 3
69115 Heidelberg, Germany

Batch number: 10607224

Printed by Printforce, the Netherlands